I W
MAKE ...

Passionate

ABOUT

Exercise

Thinking of getting this book? Read this...

The title of this book may have triggered something in you. It may have sparked an interest and made you curious enough to think, 'I need this book'. You are not alone. When I tell people what this book is all about and how it can help them, the first thing they say is, 'I need that book'.

I Will Make You Passionate About Exercise will take you on a journey with the end goal being that you will have a lifetime love of exercise. Can you imagine how your life would be different if you loved exercising? If you got to a point where your daily life involved regular activity, doing it wasn't a hard mental battle and you actually enjoyed and looked forward to it! The benefits gained by making this shift are something you can't put a price on. The physical, mental and social benefits you will experience are life changing.

This book gives you a step-by-step plan that is based on what I and my team have learnt in helping thousands of non-exercisers learn to love exercise and have it in their lives for the long term. This plan understands where you are *right now* and wisely sets you up to learn the right lessons and have the right experiences at the right time so you can be successful in bringing regular activity into your life.

Here's the problem that a lot of people have with exercise: they don't make the decision to make a change. They know they want to and maybe need to make a change but they never end up doing it. Exercise becomes that thing that they will do tomorrow, next week, next month, next year … never. Unfortunately, this means their health and fitness always comes last on the list of priorities and they continue to go down a path where nothing improves, and in fact it gets worse. Have a think right now. If you keep doing what you are currently doing, where would your health and fitness be in five years from now?

I can give you a step-by-step practical plan and wisely guide you to be successful but none of this will work if you don't make the decision to create change. You need to commit to change and prioritise yourself, your health and your wellbeing.

I have a fitness product in my local area that helps non-exercisers be successful with exercise. In one of our testimonials a lady by the name of Lizzy told us how she felt once she had committed to joining our team:

It felt amazing to join because I knew I had made a decision to change an important area of my life, and that I had a plan to get there. Instantly I knew I was putting my health and fitness first. It was great.

You can feel this way today.

You've picked up this book because it has triggered something in you. Make a decision right now that will help you feel good about yourself and will help you shift your life to a healthier and fitter place.

This book costs less than a good meal out. Surely your health and fitness is worth more than that? Make the investment now, and your future self will be glad you did!

I WILL
MAKE YOU
Passionate
ABOUT
Exercise

Bevan James Eyles

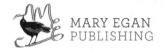

MARY EGAN
PUBLISHING

Published by Mary Egan Publishing
www.maryegan.co.nz

This edition published 2022

Produced by Mary Egan Publishing
Printed in China

ISBN 978-0-473-62139-1

To Jo, Tyla, my family, and everyone that has helped me along the way.

Contents

Introduction How my failures have led to thousands of
non-exercisers win with movement   9

Chapter 1 Get this right and you will set yourself up for
success   17

Chapter 2 The tool that will bring out the best in you   23

Chapter 3 Overcoming the biggest hurdle most
beginners trip over   33

Chapter 4 How to find a lifetime love of exercise   57

Chapter 5 The unexpected factor that delivers so
many benefits   77

Chapter 6 The number one key when setting your first
fitness goal   99

Chapter 7 What top athletes have taught me about
goal attainment   119

Chapter 8 How to get the most out of your
achievements   151

Chapter 9 How to avoid going backwards after
making progress   171

Chapter 10   When you see yourself this way you will love
             exercise forever   189

Chapter 11   The tool that will help you thrive with
             exercise for the long term   213

Chapter 12   How you can change your world in
             powerful ways   229

Chapter 13   Final words   247

About the Author   251

Introduction

How my failures have led to thousands of non-exercisers win with movement

Let's go back to 2009. I'd flown from New Zealand to Florida to present at a top fitness conference. The night before I was presenting I was sitting in my room with one of my best friends in the fitness industry, Mid Thomas.

Mid is an amazing woman who is best represented by the word 'love'. She gives so much love to everyone in her life. When Mid and I get together our conversations get deep straight away. There's no small talk, the shovels are out and we are digging into the good stuff.

This night was no different. After talking for around an hour Mid said a statement that totally changed my life. She said that we are failing with fitness.

At first I didn't know what she was talking about as in my mind we were killing it with fitness. As a fitness professional I had won my country's Instructor of the Year three times, I'd travelled the world training other fitness instructors, I was a fitness writer and podcaster, and each week I trained nearly 1,000 people in the workouts I took. On a personal level I had been a high-level

Ironman triathlete for over six years, averaging over 25 hours of exercise a week for the last ten years. Me failing, without being cocky, I just couldn't see it.

So I asked what she meant when she said we were failing with fitness. Mid replied that if we look at the stats around obesity and people's movement, more people are getting more overweight and less people are moving. If it's the fitness industry's job to help people get healthier and fitter, we are failing.

Have you ever had a moment when something is revealed to you that shows you something in a totally different light? It's like you are shown a colour that you have never seen. In this moment I saw a new colour. Mid was right, we were failing with fitness.

I have to admit that during the rest of my time with Mid that night I was a terrible conversation partner. Inside myself I couldn't let go of this idea that we were failing.

Over the next few days my mind continued to stew on this 'we are failing' revelation. As I contemplated this more and more I came to the realisation that the fitness industry sucks at helping non-exercisers and the reason for this is that fit people are designing products and programmes that appeal to people like themselves.

Think about it. One of the biggest trends in fitness over the last few years is workouts based around high intensity interval training (HIIT). Fit people love this type of workout as you push yourself to your limits and it's very rewarding when you get to the end of it, but HIIT is extremely hard. If a non-exerciser was to try a HIIT workout they would likely fail, and this is the type of exercise our industry is trying to push right now.

At this time, I had a running business that trained groups of people to run half marathons. The people doing the programme were either gym people who were already fit and wanted to run a half marathon, or they were current runners that were looking to improve their running.

I decided that I wanted to see if I could create a running product that could help exercise beginners to actually achieve a fitness goal. For the next six months I worked my butt off (and spent a lot of money) creating a beginner 5km running programme. The idea was that it would be an eight-week team training programme with coaches at every session and there would be education and support along the way.

After six months I was ready to put the programme to the market but I thought it might be a good idea to get a small group of beginners to have a trial run. I found ten total non-exercisers with a broad range of ages from 28-59 and convinced them to be in my trial crew. These were people who hadn't had an exercise routine for over ten years, had often tried and failed with exercise, and many of them were overweight.

I was pretty excited because I felt I had a programme that could change these people's lives. I couldn't wait to see all of them cross their 5km finish line in eight weeks. Unfortunately, this didn't happen. I failed them. None of them ended up running 5km.

To say I was gutted would be an understatement. I felt I had let these people down. They had taken a massive risk with me and the experience I provided them just reinforced for them that they would always fail with exercise. I felt terrible because I really did want to help these people.

While I had failed, I still hadn't given up, but I realised I was missing something. A part of my learning was to talk to all of the people in my trial group. I remember calling a lady named Sarah. When I asked her why she felt the programme had failed she said that it was just too hard.

It turns out I hadn't learnt my lesson because Sarah's comment was reinforced by just about everyone else in the group. In designing this programme I hadn't taken on board one of my revelations—even though I had made the programme easier than what I would do, it was still a 'fit person's' programme.

I knew I had to go back to the drawing board and start again. This time I did something completely different before I started. I spent a lot of time learning about the people I was trying to help. I had to understand things like:

- What insecurities do they come into exercise with?

- What barriers stop them from exercising?

- Where is their current physical conditioning at and how can I safely and realistically help them progress?

- What kind of support do they need?

- How are they different from regular exercisers?

- What would be the right level of education to give them so that they wouldn't get overwhelmed?

The list went on and on. I learnt a lot about people who struggle with exercise at this time, like:

- They can be insecure about exercise.

- They have tried in the past and have failed (often more than once), which reinforces to them that they shouldn't try.

- They find exercise extremely hard.

- Their inner story around exercise can work against them. This can be the inner voice of 'I don't like exercise' or 'I will never be good with exercise'.

- They can have issues with their bodies that can limit them with exercise.

- They don't know how to successfully bring exercise into their life.

After gaining a deep understanding of the answers to these questions and learning the lessons I learnt, I redesigned my programme. I have to admit that I was nervous when I tried it again. This time we had 30 people in the group. I felt I had made the adjustments that needed to be made but you never know until you actually do the thing. I didn't want to let these people down, I didn't want to reinforce inner beliefs that these people had around exercise that had stopped them from even trying. I wanted them to succeed more than anything I had ever wanted in my career before.

And... they did it!!! Twenty-seven of the 30 people who started this group ended up running 5km in eight weeks. The 5km run day was a highlight of my life. Here was a group of people who hadn't exercised in over ten years, had been insecure around exercise, some of them were overweight and had given up on exercise, and now they were all crossing a 5km finish line. There was elation, tears, pride, amazement, and possibility. It was a special moment in all of our lives.

In this moment I knew I had found my mission. I wanted my career to be about helping non-exercisers win with exercise. This experience lit a flame that has continued to this day.

We ended up calling our beginner running programme 'Get up to Five'. Since beginning this programme we have trained thousands of non-exercisers to successfully run 5km. We are proud of this but we are more proud of our success rate—nearly 90% of the people who join our programme actually achieve their goal of running 5km. These are people who have failed with exercise for years. In fact one of the best pieces of feedback we've had is, 'This is the first fitness product that I've signed up for and completed'.

While we love that we have helped these people achieve their 5km goal, our ultimate goal is to help these people have a lifetime love of exercise. For this reason, we created a growth pathway for our runners where they go from doing nothing to running a half marathon in a 12-18 month period (starting with Get up to Five and then moving up our product ladder). Again, we have helped thousands of people achieve this, but more importantly when people progress up this ladder they get to a place where they have exercise ingrained in their life for the long term.

In shifting the focus of my career and creating a successful programme for beginner exercisers, my team and I have learnt so many amazing lessons that are the keys to success for a non-exerciser to go from being inactive to having a long-term love of exercise, to exercising regularly because they love it, they want to be doing it and they get all of the amazing benefits that exercise can bring to their life.

This is life-changing stuff!

Why I'm writing this book and how I've gone about creating a simple system to follow so you can have a lifetime love of exercise

Hopefully by now you'll understand that I'm passionate about helping non-exercisers learn to love exercise and I'm super proud of what my running business is doing. But I want to help more people. I'm thinking if you are reading this you are probably a non-exerciser. I want to help you.

A few years ago, I wrote a book called *The Fitness Attitude*. In writing the book I wanted to give tools and strategies that can help people be successful with exercise. The book did really well and got a lot of amazing feedback from people saying how the book helped them apply these strategies into their lives. While I was happy with that book, I did wonder to myself, 'Is there a specific book I could write as a step-by-step guide that would take nonexercisers to a place where they had a lifetime love of exercise?'.

This is where Dave Ramsey came in.

You may be wondering who Dave Ramsey is? Dave Ramsey is America's number one financial content creator. His work has helped millions of people go from being in terrible financial positions to turning their lives around and being in a place where they are wealthy, or as Dave calls it, being 'financially free'.

If you listen to Dave's podcast you'll quickly understand why he is successful. He has an amazing ability to make you think, 'I can do this'. Even the person who has debt up to their eyeballs can see how they can not only move away from debt but actually be wealthy in the future.

There are many reasons Dave helps people transform their personal finances but one of the keys to his success is a formula he created which he calls his '7 Baby Steps'. The Baby Steps are actually targets you need to achieve in the correct order that if followed will guarantee financial freedom. The key to these steps is that you can't move on to the next step until you complete the step before it.

For example, Baby Step 1 is 'Save $1,000 for your starter emergency fund'. Dave explains the importance of having $1,000 saved for any unforeseen and often challenging financial events that may arise.

Under Dave's system you can't go onto Baby Step 2 until you have completed Baby Step 1. So only after you have your $1,000 saved can you then move onto Baby Step 2.

Baby Step 2 is 'Pay off all debt (except the house) using the debt snowball'. This is about removing all debt from your life in order from smallest to largest. Again, you can't move onto the next Baby Step until you have paid off all your debts (except the mortgage).

For now, I'll move on from Dave's Baby Steps. I do recommend that you check out Dave's work if you struggle in the area of finances, but you can see that what Dave has created is a clear action plan which gives you concrete targets to aim for to create financial freedom.

That's what I want this book to be; a series of steps that, when completed in the correct order, will help you build the foundation for a lifetime love of exercise. A place where exercise brings so many benefits to your life, where you are excited to exercise and where you become an inspiration for people in your life to add exercise into their lives.

Imagine how your life would be if you had this lifetime love of exercise? How would you be physically? How would you feel about yourself? What possibilities would it open you up to and what character traits would it develop? It's exciting when you think about it.

That's what I want to give to you.

In creating this book I've thought of all of the lessons and experiences you need to create success. I've determined at what stage in your journey each lesson will need to be learnt and I've put it in a step-by-step formula called the Baby Steps (thanks, Dave) so you will know where to put your focus. Most importantly every single step in this journey is believable and achievable for a total beginner. You'll see that every one of my Baby Steps has:

A Challenge: This is what you are trying to achieve when you are in that Baby Step.

The Rules: These are the criteria that you will use to help you achieve the goal of the Baby Step. The rules teach you how to set yourself up for success in each Baby Step.

Strategies: This is where I share the strategies that have been proven to work for beginner exercisers, which you will apply to massively increase your success.

Mindsets: These are the perspectives you'll use along the way. They will help you put the right thinking in place, so you are working for yourself on this journey.

Workbook: This is the planning tool you will use in each Baby Step. This practical tool will help you understand and reinforce the lessons you are learning along the way so you can cement these for the long term.

This can be a turning point in your life. You can wake up 12 months from now not only fitter and healthier but being someone who has a love of exercise and a deep belief that you will have this important thing in your life forever.

So, thanks for getting my book. Be ready to go on a life-changing journey that will end up with you being someone you may not even be able to imagine right now.

If you want to feel connected in this world you can join us at www.passionforexercise.com/social

Chapter 1

Get this right and you will set yourself up for success

Before we start 'Bevan's Exercise Baby Steps', I want to share a story with you.

A few weeks ago, I was coaching a track session with one of our running groups. This session involves our team running around a track doing different running intervals based on their current ability. I love coaching these sessions because it gives me the opportunity to be beside someone and coach them one-on-one so I can give them the feedback they need to make progress with their running.

On this particular night I was coaching one of our runners called Jo. Jo's story is pretty amazing. She joined our beginner group a couple of years ago, overweight and never having exercised before. Joining our team was a big thing for her as she had a lot of insecurities that told her she would just end up quitting—but she didn't. Over the next year Jo not only ran 5km, she ended up running a half marathon.

As I started running next to Jo I asked her how she was getting along. One thing I've learnt as a coach over the years is that if you build a relationship of trust and your people understand that you genuinely want to help them they will allow themselves to open up and be vulnerable. In this moment Jo opened up her vulnerable side to me.

She told me how she had been extremely hard on herself recently. She had been inconsistent with her training and had been making poor decisions around nutrition so she was feeling unfit and overweight. This had led her to a place where she was emotionally beating herself up. I asked Jo how much time she spends in this place where she is beating herself up. She said probably 80% of her time and I remember thinking to myself that if you are emotionally beating yourself up 80% of the time that's a tough life to be living.

After spending time gaining more understanding of her situation, I asked Jo if I could offer some advice which she gladly accepted. I gave her three tools I thought could help her get out of the place she was in. (I won't go into the details of these tools right now but you will learn these during your process of working through this book).

Once I had given my advice to Jo, I moved on and continued my coaching duties.

The following week I noticed that Jo seemed to be really focused during the track session. As a coach, you know when someone is trying to get the most out of themselves. There's a look that they have, a look of determination that is reflective of their focused inner-self. On this night Jo had that look.

After the track session had finished Jo came up to me and said that she wanted to thank me. I was in the process of saying goodbye to everyone at the session so my head was in a different kind of space and I didn't immediately click as to what she was talking about. Jo continued by saying that after last week she got out a sheet of paper and went through and applied the three tools that I had suggested to her and continued to apply them throughout the week. She said it helped her make a massive shift. She'd been on top of her exercise and nutrition, had more family time with the kids and felt like she was on the right track. She really appreciated me helping her.

I replied that it was great to see that she had shifted things around so quickly and asked how much time she'd spent emotionally beating herself up that week. She said maybe 20%.

It was so cool to hear Jo say this. What a massive shift and as a coach I wanted to see Jo stay in this healthy place so I continued by telling her how proud of her I was that she had done the work. I had given her three tools to use, she went home, did the work and made sure she continued to do it. The benefits were obvious but the real lesson to keep reinforcing is that *when you do the work you end up in a better place.*

The reason I want to share Jo's story with you is because she is an example of how when you do the work, you create shifts and if you continue to do the work, the change becomes permanent.

I imagine that you have bought this book because you want to have exercise in your life for the long term and enjoy it. I can pretty much guarantee that if you follow the steps in this book 100% you will wake up a year from now enjoying exercise. You will have it in your life regularly and it will be a fundamental part of your life, but this will only happen if you do the work.

When I was younger, I was what I call a 'content consumer' but not a 'content applier'. At the age of 20 I discovered that reading books helped me grow. I had never been much of a reader up until this point but injecting reading to my life added so much value! It made me open up to new ideas and possibilities, helped me realise my own potential and gave me the courage to try things that I had never thought possible.

After a few years I had consumed quite a few books in areas that were important to me and, while my reading was helping, I often thought when I came across another great idea 'I should do this', but once I put the book down I never followed through with action. It remained just that—an idea.

If reading was meant to be a tool to help me create change for myself, it wasn't a very successful strategy. I was learning about lots of great ideas but I was hardly ever applying them to my life and after feeling frustrated by my lack of action I decided I needed to create a better way to consume the content but then actually apply what I was learning. Here's what I came up with:

1. Use audiobooks first. When I find a book in an area I'm trying to improve in I always buy the audiobook first. Audiobooks are great because you can listen and learn while you are doing mindless activities, like housework or gardening, and you can consume a lot more content. While there's value in being able to consume more content, the real reason I choose an audiobook first is so I can determine if it's a book worth studying deeper. If I find a book that I feel will actually create change in my life, I take it to stage 2.

2. Buy the book and study it. Once I've found a book that I feel can help me grow, I buy the hard copy and delve deeper. At this stage I'll block out time in my calendar to work through the book and learn what it's teaching me to a deeper level. These might be practical tools, ways of thinking, or even philosophies that shift me. The purpose of studying the book is to create a deeper understanding of what I'm learning. From here I go to stage 3.

3. Apply my learnings. Here's where I take my deeper learnings and understandings and apply them to my life. I always aim to work time into my week where I can devote my energy to implementing them so I can get the benefits of what they can offer me.

When I added this process to my life I found I made massive shifts in myself because I no longer just thought about the idea and how I should one day do something to apply it, I actually followed through with it.

This goes back to Jo's story. She shifted because she did the work. My plan to be a content applier has allowed me to do the work in so many areas and I'm a much higher-level person because of it.

So, I want you to make a commitment before we start. I want you to treat this book like study material, commit to doing the work and trust that if you do the work you will change your life.

As we come to the end of this section, I wonder what you are thinking to yourself. What is your thinking reinforcing? Will this be another 'I should do this one day' book that you never commit to? Or is it telling you 'I'm going to commit to doing the work because I want to have a love of exercise and have it in my life regularly'. Choose the second option, it's the first step to creating any change.

Now let's get this journey started.

Chapter 2

The tool that will bring out the best in you

When I was about 22 years old I met a guy called Daniel. Daniel was one of the first people I had met who seemed to have it all together—in all areas. He was fit and healthy, had a great relationship with his wife and kids, was aligned with his culture, was excelling in his career, and always seemed to have good energy for the activities and people he spent time with. He was one of those people that everyone loved to be around.

I was fascinated by Daniel because you don't often come across people who are successful in every aspect of their life. I needed to know what he did that allowed him to manage his life so well so one Friday I was having a chat with Daniel at the gym and out of nowhere I asked him how he managed to have everything so together.

I could tell he was surprised by my question and his humble response showed the measure of the man. He said he was far from perfect and had plenty of areas to work on but he gives himself time each week to stop, reflect upon life and plan for the next week. One thing he's learnt is that when we step outside of our everyday existence and reflect, we can see what we are doing well and where we can learn and grow. So a few years ago he set up a habit of having a Weekly Meeting. He uses this time to plan his upcoming week and set up the successes he wants to experience in the next seven days.

I asked him why he felt his Weekly Meeting was so important. He said that we all fall off the wagon at times but when you have a Weekly Meeting you never fall that far; you can catch your slips and get back on track. It also helps you see how you can evolve yourself and your processes. He finds that by planning his week ahead there's a much higher chance that he will do what he sets out to do. He suggested I give it a go.

Being the keen student I was, I decided to start having a Weekly Meeting and ever since then, my Weekly Meeting habit has been one of the most powerful tools in my life.

The results are simple; when I have my Weekly Meeting my life is just better, in all areas. When I don't, there's a slippage that happens. I'm less focused, I tend to procrastinate more, my bad behaviours start to appear, and ultimately I start to get dissatisfied within myself.

After doing this for years I've learnt that my life is better with my Weekly Meeting. I've learnt that the time invested in this is paid off tenfold because when I do it I'm aligned, focused, feel I'm moving forward, and I'm able to maintain a higher level of behaviours. This experience has taught me that I'm foolish not to use this powerful tool.

There are many different ways of looking at success. One I love is 'How do you increase your percentage chances of success?'. Let's use a running example to show you what I mean.

Many people sign up for a half marathon with the dream of achieving this goal that is important to them. Setting the goal often comes with the desire to be a higher version of themselves that ends with them achieving something they are proud of.

If we look at what it takes to achieve a high level of success in a half marathon race you need to succeed in these areas:

- You need the right programme.

- You need to consistently do the training.

- You need to hit the training objectives in your workouts.

- You need to learn and practise your nutrition strategies so you are confident with them on race day.

- You need good rest and recovery strategies.

- You need to learn motivational tools.

- You need to learn how to move in the most efficient and effective way.

- You need to develop a race plan and have the ability to apply this on the race day.

While there are more aspects that I can add to this list, this is a good start. Going back to the 'increasing your percentage chance of success' way of thinking, let's say you only do one of these things—you only get the right programme. What do you think your percentage chance of ultimate success would be if you failed in all other areas? What if you got the right programme and consistently trained, do you think that would increase your chances of success? What if you did those two things well but you also nailed your nutrition, would that increase your chances of success? Obviously, the more pieces of the puzzle you can put together, the higher percentage chance of success there is.

When we are moving towards change or a challenge it's hard to 100% guarantee success but if we can do the things that increase the odds there's a higher chance that we will achieve what we desire.

One of the biggest 'percentage increase of success' tools you can use on the journey is heading your way—your very own

Weekly Meeting. If you can commit to this and create a habit that becomes a part of this journey you will massively increase your odds of success. If you get to the end of this time and you have done every Weekly Meeting I can almost guarantee that you will have achieved the goal of finding a lifetime love of fitness. The Weekly Meeting is that powerful.

How does the Weekly Meeting work?

There are a few areas that you need to get right to start and maintain a successful Weekly Meeting.

1. Set it at a time where you will be successful

In creating a habit around your Weekly Meeting the first thing you have to get right is where and when you are going to do it. This is something you need to figure out for yourself so you can set yourself up for success. The best question to ask yourself is, 'When is the best time in my week where I will have the energy, time and freedom to focus on my Weekly Meeting?'.

We are all different. You may find that Sunday night before you go to bed works best or it might be on a Monday morning before you start your week. It may be Friday lunchtime when you know you can get away from work to devote this time to yourself.

The most important thing to remember here is that you are looking for the time that will *work best for you* and will be easy to turn this into a habit.

2. Let your world know what you are doing and how they can support you

Let's say you are a busy mum and you decide that your Weekly Meeting will be at 3pm on a Sunday afternoon and you want to give yourself 30 minutes to do this. If you have kids interrupting you all the time it will be easy for you to postpone your meeting or do it in a way that doesn't actually help you. To avoid this situation, let the people in your world know about your Weekly Meeting and how they can support you.

If you are a mum, let your partner know that you need this time and work together to figure out how they can support you with this. It might be that they take the kids for some exercise or play some games with them when you are having your Weekly Meeting.

Think about the people in your world—who can help make it easy for you to start and maintain this habit? Once you have identified them, have a conversation about how they might be able to help you.

3. Create a ritual around your Weekly Meeting

A few years ago, I was working with a lady who I helped lose 30kg. While that is an amazing achievement in itself, what's more impressive is that she has kept the weight off. While there were many tools and strategies we used to create this long-term change, the Weekly Meeting was one of the keys to her success.

One day I asked her how her Weekly Meeting habit was going. She said she loves them and they are a highlight of her week. I have to admit this did sound like a bit of an overstatement as I know there is so much value in these for me so I stick to it but I have never classified it as a 'highlight of my week'.

I asked her why this had become such a significant process for her. She said she had made it a ritual: at 6pm every Sunday she makes herself a cup of tea, goes into her bedroom, puts some relaxing music on, lights some candles and then does some breathing exercises. From there she lays out everything she needs for her Weekly Meeting and goes through the process of reflecting and planning her upcoming week. At the end of it she reads some of her favourite affirmations to remind herself what's important to her. She said that if this process was going to be one of the keys to her success she wanted to create a time and space for herself that encouraged her to have her Weekly Meetings and that it was working because she loves this time.

As is often the case, my client taught me a lesson I hadn't thought of. From there, I started to put some rituals in place around my own Weekly Meeting so now I don't just do it because it's something I know adds value, I actually enjoy this time.

I want you to do this with your Weekly Meeting. Some good questions to think about here are:

- What kind of space do I want to create for myself? This can be the physical space or the kind of energy you want to be surrounded by. For example, listening to upbeat music may help you feel energised during the process.

- What can I attach to the experience that will make it more comforting? Like my weight loss client, I like to make a big cup of tea before my Weekly Meeting. There's something about having a hot drink that helps me relax and be focused. Attaching comfort to the experience makes it easier to do.

If you get these things right your Weekly Meeting will become something you look forward to and that's what this is all about.

4. Have a reflection/planning process set in place for your Weekly Meeting

This one doesn't have to be complicated. It's a good idea to have a few reflection questions such as:

- What did I do well in the last week?
- What did I learn about myself in the last week?
- Where was I off the ball last week?
- How can I improve on last week?

By thinking about these questions you can identify where you can improve. The only thing I will add to this is to think deeply about why you were either successful or not. It's one thing to acknowledge you did well with exercise because you had good energy, but if you dig deeper you can start to identify the behaviours that set you up in this place and that you want to reinforce.

For example, you could come up with a statement like, 'I had good energy for exercise because when I went to bed the night before I didn't pick up my phone. Instead, I picked up a book which was like a sleeping pill, so I got eight hours of sleep'. This statement identifies why you had more energy—you picked up the book, not your phone. By knowing this, you can reinforce this behaviour.

5. Make it a habit

Once you have all of these things in place your aim is to make it a habit. When you have had your Weekly Meeting for a while you'll understand that your life is better when you have them in place, and they will become easier, but until you get to that point it will take a bit of effort. Developing a habit is helped by having the meeting at the same time, in the same place and with the same routine every time. If you can aim to be consistent with this for two months the habit will form and it will become part of your routine.

6. Book it in your diary

This one is simple; book the time out in your diary. This is about showing yourself that this is important, and this time can't be taken away.

7. Learn and evolve your Weekly Meeting

I've given you some ideas on what it takes to be successful with your Weekly Meeting and these are a good starting point, but you want to learn and evolve your own. Aim to understand what works for you and what doesn't with the intention of learning how to get the most out of this so that your Weekly Meeting becomes more effective over time.

How the Weekly Meeting works:

Once you've found the time and place, put yourself in the right mindset and done some reflection around the previous week, then it's time to have your Weekly Meeting. This is how it works:

1. Have a weekly calendar to work with

We are all different with this one. Some of us like to use technology (like computers and phones) where others like a big sheet of paper with the week displayed like the traditional weekly planner. There's no wrong or right way, the key is to have one that works best for you. You don't want the tool to be a barrier so think about how you work best and have the tool ready before you start.

2. Set objectives for the different areas in your life

Before you block out time in your calendar you need to understand how you want to use your week. After you have done your reflection work the next thing you want to do is to set your objectives for the upcoming week. Setting your objectives is about you giving yourself focus for the different areas of your life.

In my Weekly Meeting I set objectives for the following areas:

- Music

- Business/work

- Fitness/health

- Family

- Friends

- Personal (self behaviours)

In each of these areas I give myself no more than one or two things to focus on. In any given week some of these will be big focuses and others will be smaller ones. I find that setting my objectives gives my mind a sense of where I should be thinking and when it comes to putting the calendar together it gives me a greater understanding of how I should plan my week.

How you do your objectives list is a bit like the calendar—find a way that works for you. You might buy a notebook, you might use a spreadsheet, your online calendar may even have an option for this. The key thing is to identify the different areas of your life you want to work on and set one or two objectives for each of them that week.

3. Plan your week around your whole life

One of the biggest mistakes people can make with the Weekly Meeting is to only include one aspect of their life. The whole point of doing this is to get an understanding of how your *whole* life works and where you will fit in exercise, so the Weekly Meeting clearly shows where your time will be spent from the moment you wake up till the moment you go to sleep.

4. Be realistic

I've found that when people first start implementing a Weekly Meeting they often end up only doing around 50-70% of what they have on their calendar. I think this is because when they first start they are overly aspirational with their approach. They fill it up with what they think they should be doing, not what is realistic to achieve.

Your aim is to have a calendar where you can achieve 90% of your objectives and this will happen when you have learnt what you can realistically fit into your week. The more you have your Weekly Meetings, the more you will understand how your time works and you'll get better at hitting the 90%.

If you find you are well off completing the things you planned in the first few weeks of this process don't beat yourself up! This is your calendar teaching you that you need to adjust your expectations. Learn from this and make the adjustments you need.

5. Daily review

Once you have completed your Weekly Meeting your job is to have a quick review of your objectives every morning before you start your day. Look at what you had planned for your day, then spend some time thinking about how you will complete your plan.

6. Live your day

From here, go and live your day. You will find you have a focus that helps you make better choices. This focus will help you bring exercise into your life.

Why is the Weekly Meeting so important in your journey?

When we are looking to create change in our lives we need to make sure we have both the time, but more importantly the energy, to take the actions that create this change. Too often people want to change but they never really give themselves a chance because they don't account for the time and energy it takes. This may sound familiar.

By creating this habit you will be able to plan your exercise journey in a way that gives you the highest chance of success, within the requirements of your life and those times when you have the best energy to do this.

We will do more work around this. It's where you'll learn, celebrate and plan for your next week's successes.

So, what next?

Set up your first Weekly Meeting. Remember that you are looking to get the time, place and space right both physically and mentally. You want to let your world know what you are doing and how they can support you. You want to have all of the practical things you need such as your method of calendar, a notebook, pen, and anything else you feel you need that will help (a hot cuppa?).

Read the chapter on Baby Step 1. In your first Weekly Meeting you will be starting the first step in your exercise journey so you will need to have read Baby Step 1.

I encourage you to do this as soon as possible. The sooner you get on top of this the more likely it will happen. One thing to remember is, this isn't hard. Setting up the meeting and reading a chapter of the book should take around 15 to 20 minutes. Be like Jo in the previous step: do the work, put the effort in, and you'll make the improvements.

You've got this.

Chapter 3

Overcoming the biggest hurdle most beginners trip over

Back in my early days within the fitness industry I had a client called Geoff. Geoff's first comment to me when we had our introductory meeting was that I would have a challenge on my hands with him. He said he was unmotivated, unfit, overweight and only here because his doctor said that he needed to start exercising. While Geoff said this with a cheeky smile I knew there was a lot of truth in what he was saying. Geoff was only here because he felt he *should* exercise, not because he *wanted* to exercise.

Because of this mindset Geoff wasn't too keen on spending money on a personal trainer. He informed me that he'd like to use me for a fitness programme that he could do for a month. I prefer to work with beginners at least once a week as they need more guidance, accountability, motivation and support, but this wasn't going to be the case with Geoff.

After we had done his fitness testing, I designed a very basic beginner programme for him. His current ability and motivation were very low so I needed to create a programme that he could be successful with, both physically and mentally. After taking him through the programme and giving the advice I felt he needed to get started, Geoff finished the session thanking me for my time and told me he appreciated that I had designed something he thought he could do. We booked in our second session a month from then and Geoff went on his way to start his fitness journey.

While I felt I had done my best with the time and restrictions I had with my client, I wasn't feeling confident that he would come back being a picture of success. I was right.

A month later Geoff arrived at our next session and started it with another cheeky comment, introducing himself as the Twenty Percent Man. I asked him what he meant. Geoff was a bit of a character so he laughed and said that he had managed to do 20% of what I had programmed for him but hey, it was more than he was doing before he started. He was right, this was more than he was doing before but it was hardly a roaring success.

I asked Geoff why he felt he had only hit 20% of the programme. He said it was weird because the programme I had designed for him was achievable, every time he did it he was able to complete it and even enjoy it, but other things were more important or he would talk himself out of doing it. I wanted to know more about this thinking so I asked him to expand on this. He said he would plan to do his walk in the morning but when the alarm went off he would tell himself that he could do it tomorrow. The idea of getting out of bed and sorting out his walking gear seemed impossible in that moment and more sleep was way more appealing.

As Geoff continued on with the reasons why he had only hit 20% of the programme I had an epiphany. I thought to myself, 'I've missed something here'. It was becoming so obvious and it was also obvious why I hadn't thought of this before.

When Geoff first came to see me I saw his problem as a problem with exercise. I was trying to solve the problem of how to provide a programme that was at the right level for someone who is extremely unfit. Now, if that was the right problem to solve I did a good job as the programme I designed was pitched at the right level. But this wasn't the right problem to solve.

The epiphany I had was that Geoff didn't know *how to start exercising*. He hadn't learnt how to set himself up to guarantee that he would get his first step forward with an exercise routine.

Looking back, it was obvious why I missed this at this time in my career. Exercise was easy for me. I never struggled with getting out the door to do it, it was like a subconscious behaviour. I had developed many strategies over the years and had great tools that I used which had led me to this place in my life.

I realised that the first problem I had to solve with Geoff was teaching him how to 'get out the door and start exercising'. Sure, I had designed a good beginner exercise programme but that hadn't worked because he hadn't developed the step that comes before that. No programme could work if Geoff never learnt how to *start*.

In our second session together, I decided to completely shift what I was trying to teach Geoff. I came up with a new plan, one that focused on him learning how to successfully and consistently get out the door to start exercising. This was completely different to anything I had ever done before and it didn't even focus on the exercise!

It turned out to be a total success because the next time Geoff and I caught up, the first thing he said was that he had turned into Ninety Percent Man. Geoff had learnt the most important first step in creating success for a beginner exerciser and you are about to learn this in Step 1.

Baby Step 1: Learn how to get out the door with the right attitude

When we look at people who are successful with exercise we can have a narrow view of their exercise journey. We may see photos of them finishing a fun run, hear them talk about what exercise they are going to do today or see the physical results they have achieved, but what most of us don't see is the many things they have done to create this success.

One thing that all regular exercisers are good at is what I call

'Getting out the door with the right attitude'. Before we even take the first step on a run or do the first repetition in a weights workout there are several barriers we have to overcome to even get to that place.

We have to find the right time of day to do it, have the right gear prepared and ready, plan for different weather conditions if we are training outside, and know what to do within our training. All of these are practical barriers but we also have several mental barriers. It's like there is a team of lawyers in your head and their job is to provide you with all the reasons why today isn't the right day to start, or remind you of the fear you will feel when you fail, or point out that it will be too hard. Then there is also the ever-present concern that others may judge you.

If you are going to create a love of exercise, the very first part of your journey is to learn how to be successful in doing the things that enable you to take the first step. That's what this Baby Step is all about.

The goal of Baby Step 1 is for you to learn how to navigate both the practical and mental barriers to getting started. Once you have done this step you will have learnt how to consistently get out the door and start moving because you have developed tools and strategies to help you break through these barriers.

So Baby Step 1 is to learn how to get out the door with the right attitude. To help you learn this lesson I'm going to give you your first challenge of this book:

Challenge for Baby Step 1

Get out the door and exercise three times a week, each week for the next month.

But wait...

One thing I'm going to do in each Baby Step is give you the rules, strategies, and mindsets for each of the Baby Steps. These are designed to help you make good choices and increase your chances of success within each one. It's really important that you stick to the rules as they will help this process work for you on this journey. So, before you even start thinking about getting out the door to exercise, let's look at the rules.

Rules for Baby Step 1

RULE #1: The only thing to measure is, 'Did I get out the door?'

Whenever we put energy into growing an area within ourselves, we want to see results. Results are proof that we are improving. If you start a new diet you want to see weight loss, if you study for a test you want to see you have achieved a good grade.

Whilst results are the outcome, what I've learnt is that the actual thing we should and need to be measuring is the *behaviours* that create the results. For example, if you want to lose weight, jumping on the scales shows whether you have physically achieved results but the better thing to measure is whether you planned your food well every day that week. When you measure the behaviours rather than the outcome you put your focus on behaviours that you can sustain long term. We all know that when we plan our meals we eat better, so measuring this leads you down the right path for success.

This approach of measuring your behaviour is an important part of Baby Step 1 and your entire journey. You need to understand that the bigger results are a bit further up the road. I can guarantee that if you stick to the plan in this book there will come a time when you love exercise and trust that you can have it in your life forever, but right now this isn't your focus.

A good approach to Rule #1 is to look at your thought process and actions backwards. Let's say the successful outcome you achieve is a 30 minute walk. Going from that point, work backwards and identify the steps you took to create that outcome. These could include:

1. I planned ahead and scheduled it in.

2. I let my partner know that I was getting up early so I was having an early night the night before.

3. I got my gear ready before I went to bed.

4. Before I went to sleep I preloaded what I was going to say to myself when I woke up, which was, 'Once I am up it will get easier. Get out of bed right now and enjoy that I am going for a walk'.

5. Once I was up, I quickly got my gear on, put my music on and headed out the door.

Having an understanding of each of these steps allows you to measure these things as individual wins. Rather than measuring 'Am I getting fitter?', measure 'How many times did I successfully get my gear ready before I went to bed?'.

So in this Baby Step the only thing you need to measure is, 'Did I start?' and take note of the steps you took to get out the door. If you can give yourself these ticks along the way while learning your process, you are setting up the foundation for your future.

This may come as a shock but at this stage in your journey I don't even care about what type of exercise you do. Seriously, the type of exercise isn't important. At this stage we aren't looking for a physical result. I know I'm repeating myself, but we are teaching you *how to get out the door with the right attitude.*

RULE #2: The exercise has to be easy, both physically and mentally

The lesson you are learning in Baby Step 1 is *how* to start exercising but you may be wondering *what type* of exercise to do and my answer to this is simple.

Choose an activity that you feel is easy and set it at a level that guarantees you will achieve it.

Why is this important? I imagine when you think about exercise it's not always in a positive light. You may think it's hard, that it's uncomfortable, that you will fail and so on. This thinking is working against the goal of Baby Step 1 and these feelings will make it harder to start. I want to remove this barrier from this part of your journey.

As much as you may currently have negative thoughts towards

exercise there is a level of movement that deep down you know you could quite comfortably achieve. For example, do you think you could do a very easy ten-minute walk? Or could you ride a bike on a flat road for 15 minutes? Or could you do a workout where you do one squat, one sit-up, one easy-level press-up with one minute for recovery between each move?

When I put this to you, I imagine you are thinking 'Of course I can do that'. If you are, this is the kind of level you are aiming for with this Baby Step. If my suggestions are too hard, make it easier! How about a five-minute walk?

If we go back to the challenge of Baby Step 1—Get out the door and exercise three times a week, each week for the next month—you can see how setting a level of exercise that you know is achievable makes the success of this challenge more realistic. Changing the challenge to doing three ten-minute walks each week for a month makes you think, 'I can definitely do that level of exercise'.

That's what we want.

The example exercises I shared above are on the very easy side of the exercise scale. You may know that you can do more than that amount. For example, you know an easy hour walk is well within your reach, and that is ok as well. The main thing to reinforce is that your exercise choice should be easy for you to achieve at your current ability.

Finding a level of movement that you can guarantee you can achieve, both physically and mentally, means you are setting yourself up for success in learning the lesson of Baby Step 1.

RULE #3: Don't judge the exercise or physical results

I imagine when you read the last rule you may have thought, 'What's the point of doing one squat, one sit-up, and one press-up?', or 'Ten minutes of walking isn't going to create any change'. And I'll be honest, the level of exercise that we are aiming for in this first month is not going to create any real shifts in your fitness or physical results, but that's not the point of Baby Step 1.

If your physical results aren't the point of this Baby Step but you still use them as a measure of success you are going to be disappointed and feel you are failing. When you reflect upon failure and disappointment do you find that they keep you motivated? They probably won't—they'll push you away from your journey.

If you do find that you are focusing on physical results, a good thing to reinforce within yourself is, 'When I've learnt how to consistently start exercise, I'll be able to develop my ability to exercise in ways that will give me the results I want'.

Another thing to be aware of with this rule is to never judge the exercise once you've finished. One thing I've learned in helping thousands of beginners with exercise is that they can diminish their own success very quickly. They will exercise but they still don't feel it's good enough. This triggers disappointment and failure again so in this Baby Step if you have got out the door and you have moved—you have won. Don't judge how the exercise went.

Strategies to use in Baby Step 1

Before I suggest some strategies for Baby Step 1, I want to reinforce that the whole point of this step is for you to learn the strategies that will create long-term success for you. I often think that people who struggle with exercise aren't bad at exercise, it's just that they have bad strategies.

People who are successful have proven strategies that they trust and can implement over and over again. The whole point of this Baby Step, and this book, is for you to learn the strategies that work and then to repeat them consistently till they become a habit that creates a long-term love of exercise.

With this in mind I'm going to give you strategies that I feel can help you achieve the goal of this step, but a part of your journey is to learn and develop other strategies that work for you. So add your own strategies along the way. You can even let me know your new ones that have worked for you by going to www.passionforexercise.com/social

STRATEGY #1: Plan your exercise at times that give you a higher chance of success

If we think about the motivation to exercise, a lot of people actually make it harder for themselves by increasing the level of motivation required without even knowing it! Let's look at this a bit deeper.

If you haven't exercised in a long time the first step is going to need a certain amount of motivation. But if you then decide that you are going to aim to do your exercise at 6am (and you aren't a morning person) you are now making it harder by adding another level of motivation—the motivation to get out of bed. So now you a) need to get out of bed at a time you aren't used to and b) get out the door to exercise. You can see how this approach is making it harder for you to be successful.

What we want to do is minimise our need for motivation and make it as easy as possible to be successful. Here's a good question for you to think about: If you look at your week and identify the three easiest, most realistic times for you to fit the three easy sessions that Baby Step 1 requires, when would you schedule them for?

The answer to this question will be different for everyone but it allows you to look at your week and set times and places where the need for motivation is reduced so as not to put any barriers or blocks up and it will be an easy fit into your day.

It might be that for you the easiest times will be lunch time at work because you would normally sit in the staffroom, or you know that Sunday normally means more free time and you feel relaxed on that day. It might be that you are a morning person so getting up in the morning is the best time for you.

The most important thing to understand is that you are looking to plan your three sessions at times that you feel makes it easy for you to be successful.

STRATEGY #2: Aim to keep the same times each week

When you start to plan exercise into your week you need to schedule it at the right times for what you know about yourself and around other commitments you may have. Once you've done that you want to try to create a routine so that your sessions are regular and become habitual.

Let's say you plan to go for a walk on Tuesday and Thursday at lunch time and then to do a 9am walk on Sunday. After the first week you want to repeat this routine. The more you can repeat the same times for your sessions the easier it gets to be consistent.

By the end of this Baby Step hopefully you'll find that you don't even have to think about when you're going to fit your sessions in, it starts to become a habit that routinely slots into your week. Planning and consistency is key.

STRATEGY #3: Make as many decisions as possible before the 'action' moment

The best example of this strategy is the person who packs their bag for exercise in the morning before they go to bed the night before. They are removing decisions that have to be made at the moment of action. If they don't pack their bags at night they'll have a completely different journey in the morning when they wake up. They'll have to think about what to wear, where the gear is, if they need to remember anything else for that day and so on. They are having to make more decisions which can become a barrier to their main objective which is to get out the door to exercise.

In contrast, if you wake up in the morning and everything is ready to go, you now only have one action to think about—get out the door and exercise.

The above example is a very practical way of looking at this but it can also be used with mental approaches to moments of action. One thing I have learnt in life is that the more I preload a thought or action in my mind the higher the chance I will do it. If I'm going to do a hard run in the morning, before I go to bed I will preload thoughts and visualise the actions I want to make when that moment arrives. I will see myself getting out of bed and out the door to go for this run. I will have used an affirmation like, 'You enjoy a challenge and love running when the world is asleep' as a perspective to have in place when that time hits. By preloading thoughts and actions I've found that when I arrive at the moment of action the thoughts appear and I can just get up and do what I plan to do.

So remember, your job is to create situations where you have made as many decisions as possible *before* your moment of action hits. Doing this massively increases your chances of success.

STRATEGY #4: Use 'How will I feel afterwards?' thinking

When non-exercisers think about doing exercise they often imagine that it's going to be extremely hard and this can be a massive barrier and is one of the reasons I've made Rule #2 (to make the exercise extremely easy) a key part of Baby Step 1. If we understand that thinking exercise is going to be hard pushes us away from the goal of this step, we need a great strategy to overcome this.

Before I tell you the strategy, I'm going to make a statement that is true 99.9% of the time:

No one regrets exercising once they have finished it.

The majority of the time you feel good about yourself when you have finished. Even on days where you have a bad session, you still don't regret it. Ultimately, exercise delivers a rewarding feeling at the end of it and knowing this can be used to our advantage with this strategy. Here's how it works:

If you find you are talking yourself out of doing your exercise because you think it will be too hard, deliberately catch this thinking and shift your focus away from this and towards thinking about how you will feel when you have finished. Get the feeling of how you will feel when you return from the session. Remind yourself that you will feel good about yourself and put the benefits at the front of your mind.

This way of thinking makes it attractive for you to do your

exercise because you are focused on what you will gain, and not why it's going to be hard.

This strategy is one that you'll get better at the more you practise so aim to use this in every session, even the ones where you aren't mentally struggling to get out the door. Give yourself a moment before you start and use this time to think about how you will feel when you have finished. By doing this you are installing a great habit into your exercise journey.

Also be aware of how you feel when you've finished your sessions. Start to learn how you feel about yourself, what positive self-perceptions you have, the self-talk you use, and how you feel for the rest of the day because you have done your exercise. Gaining a deeper understanding of this makes it easier to reinforce why having exercise in your day is so valuable.

STRATEGY #5: Create a celebration ritual

I'm sure my neighbours think I'm a bit weird and there may be lots of reasons for this but one of them is because when I arrive home after a hard run I always punch both arms in the air and say to myself, 'Well done, Bev.' These harder sessions deliver an emotional high for me but I also want to enjoy my effort by taking a moment to celebrate. This simple gesture of pumping my arms and giving myself praise is a little reward that I give to myself.

While we want to grow on our journey we also want to capture and acknowledge the steps along the way. I've found that many non-exercisers don't let themselves enjoy the reward of the daily steps along the way and, to me, this is doing a disservice to yourself. I encourage you to create some rituals around celebration for this Baby Step. You might follow my example and have a fist pump and praise ritual or you can create something that's more aligned to your personality.

I know that some people may think, 'Is it really worth celebrating a ten-minute walk?', to which my response is, 'Definitely!'. If you haven't exercised in a long time and you have successfully got out the door and are doing more than you have done in the past, this is a win. Celebrate it.

It is all about enjoying the process so it's up to you to develop your own celebration tools.

STRATEGY #6: Use a progress chart

When we think about motivation, one of the greatest aides is momentum. When you have maintained a new habit for a period of time you can create a sense of pride which leads to focusing on maintaining the momentum. This is where a monitoring tool like a star or progress chart can be really helpful. My wife Jo uses this whenever she's training for a running race. She will have a copy of her programme printed off and put on our fridge. Every time she completes a session she comes home and gives herself a tick on the programme. I know she feels pride in her ability to tick off the sessions and this pride and momentum is a great motivation tool for her.

Imagine you are three weeks into the challenge of Baby Step 1 and you have started and completed your exercise every time you had planned to do it. You have ticked off all of the sessions on your progress chart then one day you are struggling for motivation—do you think that looking at your chart and reminding yourself that you want to keep your momentum going will help get that session done? You probably agree that there's a higher chance if you have this in place.

Make sure you have a star or progress chart in place before you start your journey as it means you'll be building your momentum from your first step forward.

STRATEGY #7: Learn from every session

The whole point of Baby Step 1 is for you to learn how to start exercising so, while doing your sessions is the basic measure of success, the real success is learning what made you successful in achieving this. My aim is for you to create a true understanding of what you did to get started with exercise so it's important that you spend time reflecting on this.

Every time you complete a session ask yourself these questions:

- What did I do well to get started today?

- What did this session teach me about getting out the door?

- Is there any improvement I can make in my starting process?

- What do I need to do next time to create success in getting started?

It doesn't take much time to do this—you could even think about them as you are doing your stretches after your session—but spending a few minutes reflecting on these questions is going to give you massive insights into how you can be successful, and as you learn the answers you'll be able to reinforce and duplicate what works and evolve the areas that aren't working for you.

Remember, the key to Baby Step 1 is learning your strategies for success and then consistently putting them in place so this reflective time is one of the most important things you can do to ingrain these habits into your life.

STRATEGY #8: When you have bad days, don't make them bigger than what they are

One of the most important lessons I have learnt in helping beginner exercisers is that they are often walking on the tightrope of quitting early on in their journey, and it doesn't take a lot to push them off their path.

They could be doing well for a couple of weeks, ticking their sessions off, but then they have a bad day. They may not have done their session because they were being lazy, or it could be that the session they did felt like a disaster! For many beginners this one 'bad day' can trigger a response that ultimately leads to them quitting. They can emotionally beat themselves up, reinforce to themselves that they will never be successful with exercise, or even go to a place where they are destructive to themselves, which can be shown by emotionally eating or falling off the wagon.

Here's an important thing to remember—*you are going to have bad days.*

The difference between this experience for a beginner versus an experienced exerciser is that the experienced exerciser understands that bad days are just part of the game.

In all my years of exercise I've had some terrible training days. I remember one time I was running down the street so slowly when I should have been doing a hard set. I was emotionally beating myself up and there was nothing I could do to shift myself from this place. At this very moment a car with two of my training buddies drove past. I was so embarrassed. I didn't want anybody to see me in this state!

While this was a terrible training day for me, I knew that it was quite normal to have a bad day and my job was to make sure I got out the door the next day and did my programme. This one day wasn't reflective of what the whole journey was going to be like.

If you can acknowledge that you are going to have bad days— which you will—you need a plan to work through them.

Here are the steps to take on those bad days:

- **Acknowledge the bad day but also don't make it bigger than what it is:** A good way to think about this is, 'I've had a bad day today, it's nothing more than that. My job is to learn from this and put my focus on how to get back on track'.

- **Put your focus on how you make sure you complete the next session:** This is really important. While you may not have won today, you do want to make sure you win the next one. Put all your energy into making sure this happens. This will probably require a bit more effort so plan to give yourself the time and energy for this.

- **Make the next session seem as easy as possible, both physically and emotionally:** When you are planning your next session after a bad day, make the physical exercise as easy as possible. The point of this session is to get you back on track so make it easy for yourself. Doing this will make it easier for you emotionally as well.

- **Learn from this experience:** Try to learn why you had a bad day. Maybe you hadn't been sleeping enough, maybe life had been a bit stressful, or you may have pulled back on some of the tools that had made you successful in the past. While we all have bad days, we want to learn from them so instead of beating yourself up, see if you can learn from this experience so you can avoid it moving forward.

Bad days will be part of your journey so if you quit because you have one bad day you will never have exercise in your life. By learning how to navigate this you'll gain one of the most important lessons with exercise: often a bad day is followed by the most rewarding sessions. It's the ups and downs of the journey that make it so valuable and rewarding.

STRATEGY #9: Only think about the next session

Our beginner 5km running programme has taught me a lot about the mindsets and thinking strategies that allow people to be successful with exercise. Over the years I have learnt which ones are the most effective through our people who have run 5km for the first time. They tell me the messages that helped them the most on their journey and there tends to be four to six common messages that always come up.

One of these is to not look at the whole challenge but just focus on turning up and doing the next session.

This is such an important lesson to learn. Even though I've aimed to make Baby Step 1's challenge as easy as possible, if you haven't been exercising for years and I am now asking you to do

12 sessions within the next month, you could be scared off. This is because you are seeing the whole picture, which can seem overwhelming and daunting.

If you break the challenge down into small steps—which is to get out and do a ten-minute walk within the next two days—it seems more achievable. By keeping your focus away from the big picture goal and directing it towards the next small step relieves a build-up of pressure, and that helps us to be successful.

If you do catch yourself thinking about the whole challenge and feeling daunted by it, remind yourself that it's your job to put all your focus on just achieving the next session and that's all you need to do.

This lesson is one to reinforce throughout your journey through this book. There are ten Baby Steps you will work through to create your lifetime love of fitness. These are all very important for your success, but right now all you need to focus on is Baby Step 1.

Once you have won this step, we can progress to Baby Step 2. Guess what? When you are on that step that's all you need to focus on as well.

Mindsets to practise for Baby Step 1

In each Baby Step I'll give you mindsets to practise. These are ways of thinking that are designed to help you. Often our heads work against us when it comes to change, so my aim is to give you mindsets or thinking perspectives that will help you on your journey; your job is to catch yourself when your thinking is working against you and to consciously practise putting some of these mindsets in place:

- I am a beginner so all I need to do is achieve the goals and guidelines of Baby Step 1.

- Making the exercise hard is working against me. At this stage I need to keep it easy.

- If it feels hard when I'm exercising, make it easier.

- Anything more than what I did before I started this journey is a success. I'll allow myself to enjoy and celebrate this.

- All I'm trying to do right now is learn how to start to exercise.

- When I have bad days I will focus on making sure I get the next session done and making it as easy as possible.

- This is a learning experience so I'll reinforce my wins and remind myself that my job is to learn when I don't quite get it right.

- This particular Baby Step is about learning how to start exercise, so keep focussed on this.

Now it's time to start your first challenge: to exercise three times a week, each week for the next month. Exciting times!

In each Baby Step I've created a 'Workbook' section. These are designed to help you get the most out of each one. I want you to work through this workbook during your personal Weekly Meeting and design your plan for the following week. Put your rules, strategies and mindsets in place and also reflect and learn from the previous week.

This is an important part of your journey because it sets you up for success and installs the important lessons for this Baby Step.

Workbook for Baby Step 1

When is the wisest time for me to schedule my exercise during this week?

What exercise will I do? Will that feel easy for me?

How will I make sure I stay within the rules of Baby Step 1 which are:

1. The only thing I am measuring is 'Did I get out the door?'.

2. The exercise has to be easy, both physically and mentally.

3. Don't judge the exercise itself or physical results.

How do I apply Baby Step 1's strategies which are:

1. Plan your exercise at times that will give you the highest chance of success.

2. Aim to keep the same times each week.

3. Make as many decisions as possible before the 'action' moment.

4. Use 'How will I feel afterwards?' thinking.

5. Create a celebration ritual.

6. Use a progress chart.

7. Learn from every session.

8. When you have bad days, don't make them bigger than what they are.

9. Only think about the next session.

After you have completed Week 1, add these questions to your Weekly Meetings in Weeks 2, 3 and 4.

Things to reflect on:

1. What did I do well this last week?

2. What can I celebrate when focussing on learning to get out the door with Baby Step 1?

3. What have I learnt this week?

4. What is one thing that I can improve for next week?

_____

_____

_____

_____

_____

_____

Download your own workbook

With every Baby Step I have created a workbook section for you. This is designed to help you get the most out of your experience. While I have the workbook questions within this book, I have also created a completely separate workbook for you. This is a PDF or Word doc that you can download and/or print off and will help keep your work all in one place.

To get the free workbook go to:

www.passionaboutexercise.com/workbook

Where to from here?

You can go ahead and read the next chapters in the book but it's actually not needed at this stage. My advice is to put all of your focus into this first challenge for the next week or two and by the end of Week 3 you should aim to have read the next chapter but still have your focus set on Baby Step 1.

At the end of Week 3 or early into Week 4 there is some work to do for Baby Step 2—it's just some simple planning.

Success in this step equals:

- In one month from now you will have exercised 12 times.

- You will have learnt valuable lessons around how to get started with exercise.

- You will be feeling successful because you have achieved the goal of Baby Step 1.

- You will have read the next step in Week 3 of this challenge.

- You'll be ready to go onto the next Baby Step!

Imagine...

How would you feel about yourself in a month from now if you had completed 12 sessions and had followed the rules and strategies which enabled you to complete your first Baby Step? Imagine how you would feel about getting started with this journey and the excitement you would feel about the next Baby Step... it's pretty cool stuff. You are underway.

_____

_____

_____

_____

_____

_____

_____

Be supported on your journey

You are not the only person on this journey and we want you to connect with other people going through this experience. One of the best ways of doing this is through our social pages.

Once you have completed Baby Step 1 go to our social pages and use the hashtag #completedbabystep1

To join our social pages go to:

www.passionaboutexercise.com/social

Looking for a higher level of support on your journey?

Before you start Baby Step 2, I want to share something pretty special with you. It's my *Passionate about Exercise* online course.

In writing and designing this book I have created a wise step-by-step plan that will take you from doing no exercise to having a lifetime love of fitness. It will become part of your daily life and if you stick to this plan and follow the steps in this book you will get there.

At the same time, I understand that some of you may want a higher level of support and guidance on your journey, so I have created an online course to use alongside this book.

This course is designed to be a mentoring experience where each week of your journey I teach you, support you, guide you, and celebrate with you.

I've designed the course around each Baby Step and each one has its own section that you will work through. The videos and education I give you will support you throughout this journey.

The course has over 60 educational videos that have been designed to teach you the right lessons at the right times during your journey in a way that isn't overwhelming. The content in this course will ensure you avoid common mistakes and lead you along the best path towards learning to love exercise.

The course will provide you with a more immersive experience and will also:

- Set you up with a structured routine which means you are more likely to stay on your journey.

- Provide you with accountability.

- Help to remove any confusion so you know exactly what to focus on at each stage of your journey.

- Provide you with a higher feeling of support.

- Give you a deeper understanding of the lessons in this book and provide more tools that will help you to be successful.

- Help you to see your growth and make you feel amazing and proud of it!

- Enable you to make a higher-level commitment to creating change in your life.

- Help you feel part of a team as you'll connect with others that are going through the same experience.

- Help you experience a higher level of motivation.

When my aim is to achieve a goal, growth or make a change I always think to myself, 'What will give me the highest chance of success?'. This online course will provide you with a higher level of guidance which will increase your chances of having a lifetime love of fitness.

To find out more, go to www.passionateaboutexercise.com to start the online course now.

Now let's get onto Baby Step 2.

Chapter 4

How to find a lifetime love of exercise

It was one of the most confronting moments of my life. I was 24 and had just achieved the biggest goal I had ever set myself; to be an international video fitness presenter for Les Mills, one of the world's leading fitness companies.

For the past three years I had committed every part of my life to achieving this goal. I practised every day—I mean seven days a week—for over four hours each day. I got feedback from leaders in the industry, I set goals, I had affirmations which I read daily, and I continuously chased a higher level. I was obsessed.

This obsession was valuable because after three years of putting this much time and effort in I achieve something that thousands of fitness instructors desire but only a handful achieve. It was a highlight of my life but, after I achieved it, I was confronted with one of the scariest moments I had ever faced.

I remember a few days after I had completed the video work for Les Mills I got home and I felt completely lost. I was proud of my achievement but I was confronted with, 'What happens to you after you achieve the thing that you have given up everything for? What happens after that moment?'. I had a sudden realisation that in chasing this goal I had sacrificed every other area of my life. My relationship was suffering, I'd neglected many of my friendships so I felt no connection, I had fallen behind in important areas in my life (like finances), and sadly I realised that my daughter was getting the worst version of me.

I was a total success in one area of my life but if I took a step back it was quickly obvious that I didn't have much else. If anything, through chasing fitness success I was neglecting areas that I needed to develop.

This challenging personal moment made me realise that I couldn't be a one-dimensional person, that it was a dangerous place and that I needed to move away from it.

This is when I had to confront my biggest problem. I knew I needed to change my life but I didn't know how. Because I had put all of my time and energy into fitness, I had no idea of where and how I could develop myself outside of this one area, other than starting to work on my relationships. I did still love what I was doing with fitness and it was easy for me to keep doing more of it; I knew it, I was good at it, and I got plenty of rewards from it, but if I stayed where I was there were a lot of problems on the horizon for my future.

You see this problem with a lot of people who feel trapped in life. It might be a career that they get no reward from or a lack of activities that fulfil them. Often these people have a desire to find a passionate career but they don't know what their passion is so they lock in a life that is dissatisfying.

After one month of knowing I needed to change things but not actually creating any change at all, I decided I was going to have a 'Year of Discovery'. It was a simple concept; for the next 12 months I was going to try new things. There was no real set criteria for this challenge, I just had to try new activities. The idea was that by the end of the year I would have had lots of new experiences and I could then determine if I wanted to continue on with any of them.

Over the next 12 months I opened my life up to so many new things. I did some study on English writing, did an acting course, started getting piano lessons, I tried the sport of triathlon, did some travelling, and put my hand up for as many opportunities that came my way to see what life could give me.

While I generally enjoyed all of the activities I explored in that 12 months, at the end of it I had found three new passions; playing piano, travelling, and triathlons. This was such a valuable time which opened me up to developing new sides of myself but also set my life on a completely different path. Since then, I've played in bands and recorded music, seen a lot of the world, and achieved massive triathlon goals that taught me so much about myself.

I would have never got to this place or had these experiences had I not given myself the time and space to spend time discovering new possibilities.

My Year of Discovery leads towards Baby Step 2, but before we get there, I want to share a question that most fitness professionals get asked the most: What is the best exercise to do?

What do you think the answer is?

Maybe you're thinking it's something like running because it's great for cardio conditioning, developing joint strength and if done correctly can help with weight loss. I own a running business so you may think that of course I would think running is number one.

Maybe you think it's a type of strength-based exercise such as weights, some type of Strength Circuit workout, or a Pump class. Strength training delivers so many benefits for your physical conditioning and ability to function well in general life... but it's not my answer.

What about swimming? There's no impact and you get your cardio fitness using a movement that uses the whole body. Again that's not my answer.

No matter what exercise you come up with I bet you won't guess what my answer is.

If you were to ask me what the best exercise is to do, especially if you are trying to create a lifetime exercise habit, my answer would be:

The best exercise is the one you love doing.

Even if we could determine the best exercise for physical results, you would never get any results if you didn't like it, because you wouldn't do it.

When people fall in love with a type of exercise, they remove one of the biggest barriers to success. They shift from telling themselves that they *should* exercise to a place where they *want* to be doing that movement, because they love doing it.

Imagine if you absolutely loved one of these movements: running, dancing, MMA, hiking, basketball, tennis, swimming, classes at the gym, cycling (the list of possibilities could fill several pages), do you think you would be more successful at maintaining an exercise habit if you loved doing it?

While I'm sure this makes sense to you, I'm thinking that you may not have any love for one particular exercise right now. You've bought this book, so I imagine you may be feeling a bit lost on 'all things exercise'. But don't worry, Baby Step 2 is going to help you figure this out.

Baby Step 2: Spend time exploring different exercises to find the one you enjoy the most

My Year of Discovery had so much value because it gave me permission to explore without judgement. I was allowed to dip my toe into different worlds to see if they could work for me. I committed enough to have a taste, but I didn't have to eat the whole cake.

This is what we want you to do in Baby Step 2. It's all about getting out there and trying different types of exercise workouts, just to get a feel for them. At the end of this period you will have one that you enjoy the most; you may even fall in love with it. It will be this exercise that you will take with you as you move forward on your journey.

By finding the right exercise you are taking a massive step forward in your progress and you are making it easier for yourself to create a lifetime love of exercise. It's exciting.

So, what are the challenges, rules, strategies and mindsets that go with Baby Step 2?

Challenge for Baby Step 2

Over the next six weeks aim to experience between four to six different types of exercise workouts and at the end of the six weeks determine which you enjoyed the most. It's as simple as that. Experience them and get a feel for them. This is important because how do you know if you like a workout if you haven't tried it? It's this exploring stage that will help you understand what doesn't work for you, but more importantly, what *does* work for you.

You can of course choose to try more than six exercise workouts and I actually encourage it as the broader the range of experiences you have, the more likely you will be to find the one you love.

Because I want you to layer your learning experience, Baby Step 2 will sit on top of Baby Step 1. Your aim is to continue Baby Step 1's challenge of getting out the door to exercise three times a week (keeping to the rules of that Baby Step of course), but each time you explore a different type of exercise, that will count as one of your weekly sessions. For example, you may have been doing three easy walks in Baby Step 1 but now you will do two easy walks and your third weekly session is where you try something new.

At the end of the six weeks you are going to determine which one you like the most, which will be important for Baby Step 3. It will be this exercise that will become your focus for the rest of your journey.

Rules for Baby Step 2

RULE #1: Treat yourself as a beginner

For many beginners, going into an exercise environment can be scary; this makes sense as they have often failed in these environments. They can feel lost, insecure, feel they stand out and worry that they will be judged. While this mindset can absolutely be real for you, it makes it really hard to be successful with Baby Step 2—it can push you away from trying.

This rule is a bit like Baby Step 1's Rule #2; the exercise has to be easy, both physically and mentally. When you step into these environments you have to tell yourself that you are a beginner and your only job is to try the exercise at a level that feels comfortable and safe for you.

This is so important.

Let's say you try a spin class at a gym. Normally these classes can run anywhere from 30-60 minutes. That might be too much for you right now and after 15 minutes you may be finding it hard. If this is the case, get off your bike and call it a day. At this stage in the journey we aren't looking for you to complete a workout to get fitter or to be mentally strong, we just want you to get a feel to see if the workout is something that you enjoy.

To help yourself with this I suggest speaking to the fitness professional before the class starts to let them know you are new and you are just giving the workout a try and that you may leave early. You'll find that if you do this they will support you and it will be easier for you to make the right choice for yourself if that moment arises.

This beginner mindset allows you to be open to the experience and gives you permission to do it in the way that works for you.

RULE #2: Focus on what you are trying to gain from the experience, not why you don't fit into the environment

One of the biggest problems we see when non-exercisers go into exercise environments is that they are very vulnerable and can be very self aware. I remember a great example of this.

A few years ago I was talking to a lady who was a non-exerciser who matter-of-factly informed me that she hated gyms and would never go to one. When I asked her why, she told me how she had been to the gym once and when she was exercising she could see the gym staff laughing at her.

She was embarrassed and in this moment she decided that she would never go to a gym ever again in her lifetime. When she was telling me this I was ashamed of my industry and I could see why she felt this way.

Later on that day I was reflecting on this conversation as it had really affected me. As I was thinking about it I thought about everyone I know in the industry and, while as a group we are far from perfect, one thing I know about the people in my world is that we are passionate about helping people love exercise. We want to help people be successful. We don't sit around and laugh at people who are overweight and unfit, it's not what 99% of us are about.

As I thought about this I started to see that lady's situation in a different light. While I can't be 100% certain, I very much doubt that the gym staff were sitting and laughing at her. They were probably just having a personal conversation and having a laugh together between themselves. At that moment the lady, who was vulnerable and insecure in this world, saw their laughter and attached it to herself.

I could be wrong, but it can teach us an important lesson in areas we are insecure about. Often what we bring to our world will determine what we will experience from it. When you go into a fitness environment thinking everyone is looking at you in a disapproving way, you will be looking for evidence of this which you may even see when it's not there. This will push you away and make it hard for you to be successful on your journey.

A good tool to use here is called the 'spotlighting' tool. When you think about the people in your life, how much time do you spend thinking about them each day? Think about your friends and family, your workmates, and other people you interact with— how much time do you actually spend thinking about them? For most of us the answer is not a lot, and the reason for this is that we tend to spend most of our time thinking about ourselves and our own lives. It's good to understand this because you can remind yourself of this when you are in environments where you feel vulnerable, which you may do in this Baby Step.

The best perspective to take into these experiences is, 'The purpose of me being here is to see if I enjoy this type of exercise. I'm a beginner who's here to give it a try, so be kind and easy on myself and aim to be open to the workout I'm experiencing.'

RULE #3: Be open to all types of exercise experiences

It's hard to know what type of exercise you will fall in love with through this experience. Maybe you could never see yourself as an MMA fighter or you don't think you could be a dancer but how do you know if you don't try?

I'm sure through this period of time there will be some exercise that you'll walk away from thinking, 'That wasn't for me,' and that's ok, this is what this is all about. To give yourself the best chance of finding an exercise that you are attracted to, have as many experiences as possible. Dismissing exercises and movements before you even start is working against you.

If you keep focused on Rules #1 and #2 from this Baby Step and have a fun attitude towards trying new experiences you will be open to more options.

An attitude that I love to have in life is, 'I'll always give something a try'. I remember years ago I was in China presenting a high-energy physically challenging workout called Body Attack. While I was there, one of the dance instructors asked me if I would like to jump on stage with a big crew of dancers for the last track in her dance class presentation. Now, I'm no dancer—there's no way I will ever teach a dance class in my life—but in that moment I thought, 'I'll give it a try'. This led to me having one of the most memorable experiences I have ever had in my career. Being on stage (admittedly I was in the back row so not many people could see me) dancing with thousands of people in front of me was such a buzz. If I had thought, 'I'm not a dancer so I shouldn't try this', I would have missed out on a lifetime highlight.

This experience didn't lead to me starting dance classes but it made me realise that there's a part of me that does love dancing and that maybe at a different time in my life this may be a possibility I'll explore.

It's this 'I'll give it a try' attitude you want to bring to this experience. Who knows, you may fall in love with an exercise you would have never thought possible.

Rule #4: Explore movement options that have a growth/goal pathway

I love teaching a Pump class. I've been doing it for years and I think it offers a great way for people that wouldn't normally do weights to get this type of training into their lives. While this workout has a lot of value to it, it's not the type of movement I want you to explore in this Baby Step.

A Pump class is what I call a 'habit workout'. It's a workout that you do as a habit but doesn't have a growth or goal pathway. Once you have done it for a while it becomes a part of your routine and while you may get better at doing it there's no focus on progressing forward or development, it's just a habit that you maintain. This is because it's not designed this way. This isn't a bad thing, 'habit workouts' have an important place in the fitness world and in the future I imagine that you will have some workouts that sit within this place. It's just in this stage in your journey I want you to have a pathway that opens you up to goals that will develop and motivate you, moving forward.

This is not to say that you can't try gyms; you just want to look for options within a gym environment that has a growth/goal pathway. This could include body building, power lifting, strength challenges Games, or a product that personal trainers or gyms can provide.

The other valuable part of finding an environment that has a growth/goal pathway is there is often infrastructure in place to help people move through the system and experience continual growth. Think of the belt system in fighting sports. The leaders in these worlds are working to a model that helps manage your growth and gives you the next stages as you experience success.

So when you are exploring what movements you are going to try make sure you identify the ones that have a clear pathway for growth. This will help you a lot when we get to Baby Step 4.

Strategies to use in Baby Step 2

STRATEGY #1: Brainstorm ideas

This strategy is pretty simple. When you first sit down to plan the exercises you are going to explore, grab a piece of paper and brainstorm all of the different exercises you are going to try. This Baby Step goes for six weeks so remember, at a minimum you want to experience four to six different types of exercises but at this stage just write down all of the ones that you think you *could* try.

Once you have done this, rank the ones that appeal to you the most. From there you will commit to your top six.

The only thing I would add to this is try and mix the experiences up. Think of creating a diverse range of options that will give you many different experiences like playing tennis, trying boxing, going on a walk with a tramping club, trying a team sport and so on.

STRATEGY #2: Be an amazing planner

Your organisation around this Baby Step needs to be top notch. Each week you will be going into a new exercise world and you want to make sure you set yourself up to be as relaxed as possible when you are there. If you turn up late, are flustered and confused, it's not going to be a good experience. Great planning helps you to avoid this and puts you in a state where you can be more open to the experience.

To achieve this you want to know and do these things:

- The location and how long it will take for you to get there.

- How the carparking and transportation to get there works.

- How long you need to be there beforehand.

- What gear you'll need for the workout.

- Whether they have options for first timers.

Having knowledge around this will give you the best chance of turning up in the right emotional state to be able to get the most out of the experience.

STRATEGY #3: Introduce yourself to the instructor or fitness leader and tell them that you are new

As I mentioned earlier, the fitness programme I'm most known for in the Les Mills world is Body Attack. This is a high impact, very challenging workout. The worst experience I can have when I'm teaching this class is to turn around after I have put the music on and see someone who is totally new in the room, looking like they are out of their depth. While I try my best to safely help them through the workout, deep down I know that this probably isn't a good experience for them and there's a high chance they won't come back.

These situations are rare because I'm normally there well before the class begins and I make sure I identify new people so I can have a chat and help them understand how they can be successful with their first experience. I let them know how to use options to keep the intensity manageable, give them permission to just try half the class and teach them anything else they need to know before we begin.

Introducing yourself to the instructor and letting them know you are new and very much a beginner is so important. This enables them to give you the key information you need, tell you how you can keep the workout at beginner level, and they'll keep an eye out for you.

The most important point of this strategy is that *you need to lead this*. While great instructors will be there early and will probably

67

see that you are new and approach you, not all instructors will. That's why you have to take control of this for yourself.

I understand this will be tough for some people as it can be a vulnerable place to be in and if you do feel this way, remind yourself that if you build a connection with the instructor before the experience you massively increase your chances of a successful experience. Also remind yourself that they are only human and they probably want to help you love the exercise they are instructing.

This strategy reinforces Strategy #2—be an amazing planner. To meet the instructor/fitness leader you have to be there early and great planning is key to this.

STRATEGY #4: If you know someone who already does this type of exercise, go with them

You may have a friend who's in a running club that has an entry-level programme. A good strategy is to ask them if you can go to the session with them. Sure, they may be more experienced at running, but the thing to remember is people want to sell their exercise drug. Think about the people in your life who exercise regularly, and I imagine they have a type of exercise they are passionate about. You'll see it in their social media feed; they post about their 'exercise fix'. The thing is, these people want more people to have the same passion and that's what I mean about them selling their exercise drug, they want others to experience what they love.

I guarantee a running friend would be over the moon to get you along to their running group to try it out. It means you are experiencing their passion and by going along with a friend you break down a lot of barriers. They will teach you what you need to know, the type of language used in this world, introduce you to other people in the group and make you feel welcome. This person is a powerful ally to have on your side. If they are a friend you feel you can share your insecurities and vulnerabilities with leading into this, although it may be scary to do so. Allow them to support you through this experience.

STRATEGY #5: It's ok to leave if it's just not right for you, but don't make this the norm

In the sport of Ironman triathlon, professional athletes are at risk of creating a dangerous habit that can limit their career. It happens when they are in a race and it's not looking like they are going to get the result they want and at this time some athletes decide to withdraw from the race.

There is some logic to this; it's their job to get results and if they don't get results they don't make money. It's understandable to think that if they aren't going to make money they are best to pull out of the race and focus their energy on the next event and hope to do better next time, but this can have negative consequences.

These athletes lose opportunities to gain mental toughness. If they get into the habit of giving themselves the option of quitting, they risk developing a habit that will appear in that moment when they need to be at their best. When the going gets tough or there are barriers ahead of them, if they are used to giving themselves the option of quitting, they often don't have the mental edge to push through that moment, which leads to a weak performance. You tend to see the greatest Ironman athletes will always finish a race, even on days where they underperform, and doing this is more about 'being an athlete that doesn't give up' than anything else.

You might find that in one of your experiences you just aren't enjoying it or it's just not happening for you. In this moment I would encourage you to continue through to the time frame you gave yourself and not quit. While you may ultimately decide that this experience isn't going to be one that you want to do long term, there will be some lessons that you will learn from it.

If you definitely feel you need to leave, then do. In situations where you don't feel safe, if you feel extremely vulnerable, or you feel you may get injured, of course put yourself first, but if you are sitting on the fence about leaving early, I encourage you to stay to the end.

STRATEGY #6: Reflect upon every session

The whole point of this Baby Step is for you to experience movements and activities that will help you find one that you could love and for this reason it's really important to do some reflection after each experience you have. Here are some great questions to explore around this:

- What did I like about the experience?
- How did I feel during and after the workout?
- Did I enjoy the movement?
- Where did I struggle?
- Do I want to do this again and ultimately make this a movement that I will commit to for the long term?

Aim to go through these questions as soon as you can following the completion of your experience. You can write them down if that helps but you want to have a clear understanding of where the experience sits within your overall scale of enjoyment.

STRATEGY #7: Even if you find the movement you love first up, keep exploring other exercise options

Harry Potter fans, prepare to be slightly offended. A good friend of mine is an English teacher. He's one of those teachers you could make a movie about. He uses his passion for English and teaching to transform the lives of the kids in his world of education.

When the Harry Potter books were in their peak of popularity my friend and I were talking about why they were so successful with adult readers as well as younger readers. He made an interesting comment about how they're good books but he thinks the main reason they are popular with adults too is because they are the first books they have read in years. It's probably not so much that Harry Potter is the most amazing series of all time, it has just reminded these adults how much they love reading.

Leaving the discussion around the merits of the Harry Potter story out of this equation, he had a point. Reading can be lost as we get older and we have more limits on our time, but when we do read we often find it so valuable and we really enjoy it, we are reminded that this is something we should be doing more of. This point is also one to be aware of in this Baby Step.

You may go along, try your first exercise from the list you brainstormed and get the most amazing high. After this you may think to yourself, 'I've found the one. There's no need to continue with this Baby Step as I love this!'. This may be the case. It may be the one, or it might be that you are just like the adult reader who picked up a book for the first time in a long time and you are just getting an 'exercise high'—something that you haven't felt in a long time.

As you progress through your journey, it may be that the first movement you try in this Baby Step is the one you fall in love with and that would be great! But even so, I want you to keep exploring the other four to six exercises you had on your list. If you find 'the one' in that first experience, the other experiences will just reinforce this so there will be great value in seeing them all through.

STRATEGY #8: Accept that there is a cost involved and see it as an investment

A few months ago, I was talking to a guy about my running group. He hadn't exercised in years and was feeling dissatisfied with where he was with his health and fitness. The more I told him about what we did the more his eyes lit up and I could tell he was getting excited about the prospect of bringing exercise back into his life. He asked me how he could get involved so I told him to go to our website, pay and register for the team and he would be all set to go with the next group.

Suddenly there was a total shift in his energy, it was like he was offended by the fact we charged for our service. I told him it will be the best investment he can make in himself as he will be improving his health. He said sorry but this wasn't for him and he made it pretty obvious that this conversation was over.

Now, I don't know if this man ever went on to exercise but it's probably unlikely. Unfortunately he didn't see spending money on his health and fitness as an investment.

While you may be able to get a free trial at most places you explore exercise, at some stage there will be a cost involved. I understand that for some people this can be hard to get your head around but try to shift your thinking from this being a cost to seeing it as an important investment in yourself.

Let's say this exploratory period costs $150. Would finding a lifetime love of fitness where you get to experience so many amazing physical and mental benefits be worth that much? To me, $150 to change your life is the best use of your money.

By seeing this as an investment in your health and wellbeing you'll be removing a barrier that could otherwise hold you back.

STRATEGY #9: Work around any limits you have

Some beginner exercisers will have real limits they need to work around. It could be that they have an injury or excess weight that limits certain types of movement. It's important to acknowledge that this is real and if you find yourself in this situation certain types of movement may be out of the question.

The only thing I would say here is look to see if there is an option that could work for you. Sure, you may have to walk with the running club or you may have to do bodyweight squats instead of bar squats in a strength style of workout but there may still be a level that could work for you. That's the great thing about movement; there are options that can work for all types of people. Allow yourself to do what's right for you but be open to working with options that will provide more experiences.

STRATEGY #10: Determine which exercise you like the most

At the end of the six weeks you will have had four to six different exercise experiences. You'll probably find that there were some that you realised pretty quickly weren't for you, there may be one or two that were fun but you could take them or leave them, and there will be one that you enjoyed the most and want to try again.

Finding 'the one' is the whole purpose of this Baby Step. It's going to be the movement you will commit to as you move into Baby Step 3.

Hopefully, at the end of the six weeks the answer will be clear, but what if it's not? If you have two that shine out from the rest, you can pick either one of them. Go with your gut on this, you may want to think about the long-term commitment you are going to make and determine which one is the most appealing based on that. Ask yourself, 'If I'm going to commit the rest of my journey to this movement, which one do I like to do the most?'

What if you haven't found 'the one'? Give yourself a few more weeks in this Baby Step and try a few more experiences. If you find yourself still searching, that's okay! Stay committed. We can all lose our mojo if we don't get to where we want to get to within the time frame but stick at it, you will get there.

If you feel you just can't find your favourite, go with what you instinctively feel is the best of what you've tried. You're going to see that the next stage in your journey adds so much more than just the movement you pick. Sure, finding the right movement helps, but there are other more important factors that will create your lifetime love of exercise.

Mindsets to practise for Baby Step 2

- I'm a new person in this area so I'll treat myself like a total beginner.

- When I go and experience the exercise I'll allow myself to take it as easy as I need to.

- The purpose of this is for me to try different types of exercise so I'll go into each with an open mind.

- I'll keep my focus on how I can get the most out of the experience when I'm in it.

- I'll see the enjoyment every experience has to offer.

- If I have one bad experience, I will continue on with the next one.

- I'll plan like a legend so I can give myself the highest chance of success.

- This Baby Step is important in my journey to find a love for exercise.

Now it's time to start Baby Step 2.

Here is your workbook for the next six weeks. This will help you get the most out of this Baby Step and by the end of it you'll have found a movement you enjoy and will take with you into the next stage.

Workbook for Baby Step 2

1. How do I make sure I keep the lessons from Baby Step 1 in place throughout this week?

2. When will I do my brainstorming session?

3. What new exercise will I be trying this week?

Things to consider before your next exercise experience:

1. What planning do I have to do to make sure I have the best experience possible and how can I make sure I get there early to meet the instructor?

2. Is there someone I already know who does this exercise that I can go with?

3. How do I make sure that I treat myself like a beginner when I'm there?

4. How do I focus on what I am trying to gain from the experience, not why I don't fit into the environment?

5. What perspectives will allow me to make the most out of this?

Things to reflect on after the exercise experience:

1. What did I like about the experience?

2. Were there things I didn't like about it?

3. Is this a movement I would like to explore further?

4. Are there any thoughts I want to remember about this?

5. Do I feel good about myself after doing this?

6. Any other comments

Repeat this process for all your Weekly Meetings in this Baby Step.

Where to from here?

Baby Step 2 starts from here. You should be reading this towards the end of Baby Step 1 so in your next Weekly Meeting you'll do your brainstorming and planning for your first exercise experience to try.

By the end of these six weeks you should have your preferred movement. This is the one you will be taking with you on the rest of this journey. In Week 5 come back and read the next step as you'll need to do some planning for that Baby Step.

Success in this step equals:

- You have maintained the lessons you learnt in Baby Step 1.

- You have tried between four to six different exercise experiences.

- You have applied the rules, strategies and mindsets from within this Baby Step.

- You have one favourite exercise that you will take with you on your journey.

- You'll be ready to go onto Baby Step 3!

Imagine...

If in six weeks from now you had discovered a type of exercise that you enjoyed, that was appealing to do, and that you wanted to go back and do again, imagine how this would shift how you feel about exercise and this journey as a whole.

Exciting stuff. It's time to start the journey of Baby Step 2.

Be supported on your journey

Once you have found the movement you enjoy the most go to our social pages and share it with us.
Use the hashtag #foundmymovement

To join our social pages go to:
www.passionaboutexercise.com/social

Remember you can sign up for the Passion for Exercise course by going to:
www.passionaboutexercise.com/course

Chapter 5

The unexpected factor that delivers so many benefits

When I first started in fitness, I was hungry for success. This hunger triggered a work ethic that I didn't know existed within me and it created a desire for learning. I became a sponge for any type of book that I felt could help me grow.

While I read all types of books, at that time I was reading a lot of self-help books. After a while I realised that most of them have the same messages, one of these being, 'Learn from those who have been successful in the area you want to succeed in'. I took this message on board and applied it to an extreme level. I wasn't shy in approaching anyone that I thought could guide me and luckily so many people were generous with their time and energy and quite happy to help me.

In the area of fitness there was one person who I really wanted to learn from, a lady called Sue. She was the top fitness professional in the country and was successful in all areas a fitness professional could be judged on. She had a profitable business, massive name recognition, was a role model with her own fitness but most importantly she had a phenomenal ability to help huge numbers of people to achieve fitness goals.

I really wanted to meet up with Sue but there was a problem, she lived in a different city. These days that wouldn't be a problem as we could jump on a video call but back in those days we didn't have that option. Eventually I was heading to her city to do some work so I got in contact with Sue and asked if I could shout her a coffee so she could share some insights that could help me. She agreed.

In my mind I had one hour to learn from the superstar in my game and I wanted to make sure I made the most of this opportunity.

Have you ever heard the saying, 'Don't meet your hero because you will be let down?' Well, this meeting was an example that completely disproves that. Sue was everything I'd hoped she could be. She was friendly, encouraging, and generous with her insights. I could have spent eight hours with her and it still wouldn't have been enough time.

More than any other thing in my career, that one hour with Sue had the biggest influence on me. What I learnt in that hour guided everything that I have done since.

I clearly remember her saying that people want to belong. They need a sense of purpose in their life and they need to grow. Fitness is a great way to provide all of this. Sue had always seen it as her job to be a creator of a world where people have these things and she uses exercise as a way to give this to them.

I can't remember word-for-word the rest of our conversation, but I did take notes and here are the bullet points from my time with Sue:

- Our job is to create a community that people can attach to, that helps bring meaning to their lives. Part of them being in a community means they help improve others' lives as well as their own. Think long and hard about what type of community you are aiming to create and lead it in a way that allows people to thrive.

- We need to understand the different needs of our people and help guide each individual in the wisest way for them. Some will need tough love, some will need support, some will need to be challenged and some will need positive reinforcement. A one-size-fits-all approach doesn't work. Become a master of learning how to guide each individual.

- Be like a dog. This one makes me laugh, looking back on this conversation. When you hear this you could take it many ways. The way Sue described it to me was one of the best things about being a dog owner is that your dog is always happy to see you. When you come home from a tough day at work your dog responds to you like it's the best moment in its life. As a fitness professional, your people want that from you. They want you to be happy that they've turned up so always give them the energy that makes them want to come back.

- Never forget that your job is to help them grow. While there are many benefits for having fitness in your life, ultimately people invest in you to help them create change and get results. You may offer so much more than the physical benefits but never forget that you have to continually help them grow.

You can understand why my time with Sue was so valuable. Her insights have massively influenced how I have built my career and even to this day I challenge myself to evolve these even more.

Soon, I'm going to share with you why Sue's lessons are so important for Baby Step 3 but before I do I have a question for you.

What's one area in your life that you have succeeded in?

It might be your career, playing an instrument, leading other people, or even cooking. Think of one area right now. If you were to work with a total beginner who really wanted to achieve success in this area, would you just give them an app and leave them to it? Of course you wouldn't—there's a high chance they would just fail and there is a reason for this.

When we are working in an area that is new to us there are so many lessons we need to learn, both through succeeding and also through making mistakes. If we want to take the wisest path forward the best thing we can do is get great mentors around us, mentors who have 'been there and done that', have learnt the lessons through success and failure and more importantly that they have the knowledge of how to guide someone at our level.

One of the biggest mistakes beginner exercisers make is that they try to do it all by themselves and this is a recipe for disaster. There are so many hurdles to overcome before we have success and often beginners don't see them coming, and when they hit them they don't know how to respond and overcome them. Fitness apps that give you a programme are a great example of this. So many beginners download these with good intentions but they never achieve the goal. Maybe you have been one of these people.

There is a very popular app that beginners use to start their journey towards running 5km. I once read that only 1.86% of people who download the app end up actually running 5km and this is the ultimate definition of failure! Only 1.86% succeed! These people download the app dreaming of running 5km but within weeks the app just represents another fitness failure in their life. While the programming within this product is pretty good as a fitness plan for beginners, there are so many other lessons people need for success, lessons that a wise mentor can help them learn.

It's this simple, if you want to succeed with exercise you have to put the right people in your world and with this in mind I want to introduce Baby Step 3.

Baby Step 3: Find and commit to the right exercise world for you

Up until this point in the book you have learnt how to get out the door with the right attitude (Baby Step 1) and then you have spent time exploring different types of exercise and have found the one you enjoy the most (Baby Step 2). These steps are important in your journey and may be the hardest as they are very self reliant, but to me Baby Step 3 is the most important step of all.

The purpose of this step is for you to *find your exercise world*. To find the people who will guide you, support you, become your friends, give you purpose and help you make the inner shift from being a non-exerciser to being someone who sees themselves as a fit and healthy person. If you can find the right exercise world for you, exercise becomes easy because that world will be a place that you want to be in. If it's attractive you'll want to spend more time there. You won't need to find motivation, you'll have it in spades.

Challenge for Baby Step 3

Over the next four weeks explore as many different providers in your chosen movement as you can.

Unfortunately a lot of people put convenience first on their list when they are choosing exercise providers. This does make sense—if you join the gym that is a two minute drive from your home you'll have no excuse not to go. The problem is, convenience is not a motivator.

In finding your fitness world you need to find your 'attractive place', the environment that brings out the best in you and creates a desire to be there more often. When you find this you won't mind driving 20 minutes to get there because when you are there it's amazing in every way.

Over the next four weeks try as many of the providers of your chosen movement as you can because by the end of this Baby Step you will commit to one of them—the one that is best equipped to help you fall in love with your exercise.

Before we get into the rules, strategies and mindsets for Baby Step 3 I want to teach you what to look for when you go and experience the different providers. You need to look through a lens that will help you make the best choice around committing to your fitness world.

There are three areas I want you to be ultra aware of when you visit the different exercise providers.

1. They have to have amazing leaders/mentors

The reason Sue was the one person I wanted to learn from in the fitness industry was because she was phenomenal at changing lives. If you lived in Auckland at that time and asked me what would be the best thing you could do for your fitness my answer would have been to go and work with Sue.

Based on the lessons she taught me, you can see why I would say this. Getting Sue on your side massively increased your chances of success. She was a leader who knew how to get results out of her people and that's the type of person you need on your team.

When you are creating your fitness world look for the type of leaders who have the ability to help people actually achieve their goal. These are some things to look for in your leaders:

They need to know their stuff: This one is pretty basic. They need qualifications in the area that you are trying to improve in. With fitness this can be a problem in today's world of social media. There are many people who have massive followings because they look amazing but they don't even have the basic fitness qualifications. It's one thing to have a good body but to help others you need qualifications. Make sure the leaders you choose have these.

They have experience in the area you are looking to grow in: Let's say I want to run a half marathon—I wouldn't go to a bodybuilding personal trainer to do this. If the bodybuilding personal trainer was qualified they would probably have a basic understanding of the principles of fitness but no experience in the area I want to achieve my goal in. Qualifications are important but specific experience is just as important. Choose people who have 'been there and done that' in the areas you are looking to achieve in. By getting these people on your side you are getting experience and knowledge that will increase the chance of your success significantly.

They have a proven track record of helping people just like you: This is a biggie. When I shifted a big part of my career focus towards helping beginners learn to love exercise I realised that the lessons I had learnt about how to help people be successful with exercise didn't work with these people. Ninety percent of the people I had worked with up to that point were fit people and I quickly discovered that I needed to learn a whole new set of lessons in how to help beginners.

I'll admit that at first I didn't always get it right and some of the beginners I first worked with I failed with because I was still using my 'fit people' thinking. But as time went on I learnt a completely new way of thinking and strategies to use when it came to beginners. Now I can proudly say that I can confidently help a beginner learn how to be successful with exercise.

There are a lot of fitness leaders who have only ever worked with people who already have an exercise habit or are already fit, and while these people do important work, when it comes to choosing your leaders make sure they have a proven track record of helping people just like you—and not just once. Do your research. Ask about their qualifications, their experiences and get testimonials from people who they have helped achieve big fitness goals. The effort you spend here will have a massive payoff on your journey.

2. There has to be a community

One of the proudest achievements of my fitness career is the success of our beginner 5km running group, Get up to Five. Our target market is people who haven't exercised in over ten years, are unfit, often completely inactive, maybe overweight and are unconditioned. These people are the ones who have failed so often with exercise that they have completely given up.

Since starting the programme we have trained over 4,000 non-exercisers to run 5km. The app I was talking about before has a 1.86% success rate and we have an 89% success rate. That's right—89% of these unfit, non-exercisers actually run 5km with us. We are so proud of this.

There are many things we do to create success for our people—wise programming, amazing coaching support, education, and providing the right level of motivation at the right time—and while all of these things are so important for their success, when we ask our people what was the number one key to them running 5km, none of those answers are given.

The answer we get every single time is 'the group'.

The magic of Get up to Five is that you are joining a group of people who are all of similar ability and are all working towards the same goal. When you have a shared experience, where you are growing in important ways with a group of people who are all on the same journey, something special happens.

Whilst the Get up to Five programme and structure is vital to the success of our runners, we also understand that if you can have great relationships within your exercise environment, people will keep coming back and we do a lot to facilitate this between our runners. An example of how we do this is when we train our coaches we guide them how to create connections between people, and at our introduction seminar we do group work that is all about establishing relationships.

The fundamental intent around everything we do is, 'How do we build and deepen the relationships between our runners?'.

I'll say it again—the number one key to success for our runners is *the group*. One of our runners, Lisa, said in a testimonial she gave us: 'By the end of the first session I knew I belonged'. This is what community is all about.

There are four areas to keep in mind when you are looking for a community:

What is the culture/philosophy of the community? This is important to understand. Culture and philosophy are the undercurrent of any community. They will guide how choices are made and how people will behave. The way I like to think about this is, the culture and philosophy subconsciously guide how I act towards myself and others within the community.

With my running business, our runners quickly learn that

we are a group that encourages everyone's growth, that we all support each other and we have a lot of fun along the way. We don't have to tell our runners this. When they come into our world they pick up on it and because our culture is strong they show this side of themselves to the rest of the group.

When you are exploring your exercise groups try to get an understanding of their culture/philosophy and see if it feels right for you.

Is everyone treated the same? In every exercise community there is going to be a wide range of abilities but how each individual is treated should be the same. The support, guidance, and opportunities that are provided should be the same for everyone.

Is it fun? Often people are scared of exercise because they are worried about how hard it will be and are concerned about a possible 'drill sergeant' environment and being yelled at. I have nothing against this approach. It can be successful for people at a certain level but when you are at the beginning of your exercise journey a fun environment is much more appealing.

This doesn't mean that there won't be tough times in your training—there will be—it's just that the general feel of the environment needs to be one of support. 'We are going to have fun while we are together' is the vibe you want. An environment that provides laughs along the way is one that is more appealing to return to.

Does it make you feel like you are part of a team? Humans want to belong to something. The massive success of CrossFit is a great example of this. CrossFit gives people a sense of belonging to something bigger than just a workout, so much so that it's known as a bit of a cult to those not in the CrossFit world.

While many are critical of this, to me, this is a total success in fitness. I've never been a CrossFit exerciser but the people I know who are have reached higher levels of themselves through this product. They feel part of a team and because of this they are more committed, achieve more, and have a sense of belonging with the other people in their CrossFit world.

The great thing is, there are many fitness groups within all types of movement in every community throughout the world where they have achieved the same sense of belonging. Sports clubs, running groups, amazing gyms, tramping groups, dance schools, the list goes on and on.

In the area of movement that you have found in Baby Step 2 there will be a community of people who will make you feel you belong. When you find those people you have found one of the most powerful motivators for you to change your life. It's these people who will become your friends, who you'll have amazing life experiences with, who will support you, and who will help you love exercise for the rest of your life.

3. They need to have a level that is achievable for your ability

When I started my running business we started with a half marathon group. At that time I loved the idea that we would be able to help all types of people run half marathons, however I quickly discovered that we were only helping two types of people; runners who were looking to get faster or fit people who were looking to get into running.

After being frustrated that we weren't helping beginners I realised there was more we needed to create. I remember going for a walk in the hills one day with my wife Jo and saying that we need to create pathways for growth so we can take someone who is doing absolutely nothing right now and get them to run a half marathon in a year to 18 months. This is when we created our growth pathway which works like this:

Beginners start with Get up to Five. This is designed for completely new runners with the focus being on safely conditioning them to running, helping them build their exercise habit, building connections, and keeping the environment safe and supportive.

Once they run 5km they do our Return to Get up to Five programme. This programme gets them to run 8km, it adds beginner intensity into their running but we leave it as a self-guided experience with our coaching team on hand to help them explore this.

86

From there they step up to Club10k. By this stage they are physically and mentally ready to develop intensity into their exercise. We start to push them but we do it in a careful way; we are teaching them about intensity and how to bring it into their running. At the end of this programme they can run 10km and have a good base and understanding of intensity.

The last step is RaceTeam, where we take them to their half marathon finish line. This is our most advanced programme where our runners are treated like athletes. There's a higher expectation on them and the training demands are more at the top end.

As you can see, what we have created is a development pathway for runners. We have options for all levels. Beginners can safely slot into Get up to Five and the athletes can do RaceTeam. When people look at our products they can see that there is something for them, no matter what their current ability is.

This is what you need in your exercise world. We know that you are exploring at a beginner level right now but the community you find in the movement you like should have something like our Get up to Five.

Unfortunately, not all fitness worlds will have a clear pathway for growth but this doesn't mean you should instantly give up on it. Have a talk to their leaders and see if they can cater to your level or modify their products to work for you. Who knows, you may open them up to creating products for people at a beginner level if they don't cater for them currently.

When you find a world that understands and can cater for you right now, there will be a much wiser pathway for you to walk down which will massively increase your chance of success.

Rules for Baby Step 3

RULE #1: Give every place a try

Let's be honest, many of us can judge a book by its cover or can be attracted to the shiniest thing, but this can lead to us dismissing otherwise valid options that may not have the biggest marketing budget. In this Baby Step I want you to be mindful of this. Your job is to try out as many of the facilities that provide the movement you like. Approach this with a 'Don't judge until you've experienced it' way of thinking.

There's a high chance that this will lead to you having some average experiences but it will also help you figure out which fitness world will suit you best. We've all experienced the company who is good at marketing but doesn't deliver on their promise, or the company that's hopeless at marketing but has an amazing product and customer experience. By the end of this time you will actually know which providers will have the highest chance of helping you to create a lifetime love of exercise.

What do you do if you live in a place that has too many options? Get around as many of them as possible but if there are just too many, aim to try a variety of the options available. Let's say you have discovered that you love group fitness classes and you have a lot of gyms to choose from. Aim to try a variety of the big chain gyms as well as the smaller and the boutique offerings. This will give you a wider sense of what's out there.

What if you live in a place that only has only one option? This is a bit more challenging but some of you will experience this. If you are in this situation you need to build a relationship with the leaders in this environment. Let them know that you are on this journey and that you'll need an offering that will work for you. You may even want to suggest that they read this book so they can get an idea of what you need. If you communicate your needs and goals well they should be able to provide what you need.

RULE #2: Accept there is a cost but see it as an investment in yourself

I know I touched on this in the last step but it needs to be reinforced again. For you to create a lifetime love of fitness there is going to be a financial cost. I understand that there are people who genuinely can't afford to pay for exercise providers but in the grand scheme of things it's a small percentage.

I remember someone once asked me if my spending on myself represented what I feel is important to me. This is a great question to explore. Many of us express that certain things are important to us but when we look at our actions they don't align. In committing to the journey in this book you are saying that you want your health and fitness to be important to you and if this is the case there will be a financial cost.

In a testimonial that a lady called Teresa did for us after she had completed our Get up to Five programme, she said, 'We spend money on food, coffees, clothes and other things that aren't that important. If we can't spend money on our health and fitness, what are we doing?'. This statement is so true. Often we do have the money, we just need to pull back on less important things and put it into investing in ourselves more.

I guarantee that as you start walking down this path towards developing a lifetime love of exercise this will be the best investment you make in your life. So don't resist having to pay for your fitness experience, but do make it work within your budget and embrace that this is an investment in you and it will be removing another barrier to your success.

One quick point: In Baby Step 3 you may be able to take advantage of free trials with some providers. Unfortunately, the ones that charge a one-off fee for a class or session are often the most expensive option. Be aware of this and know that initially this may be the most expensive time in this discovery phase but once you find the community you want to get involved with, having a longer term commitment will almost certainly be more cost effective. Do your best to ask for free trials but also understand that the investment you make right now is really important because you are better off to spend a bit more to find the right world for you as you start out.

Strategies to use in Baby Step 3

STRATEGY #1: Use the tools you used in Baby Step 2

At this point there is crossover with the rules and strategies you used in Baby Step 2 and while this part of your journey is specific to the movement you enjoy the most, it is still a time where you are trying out different worlds. Baby Step 2 may have built up your confidence by putting you in different fitness environments but you still want to keep on top of how you approach this time.

Here's a recap of the rules and strategies from Baby Step 2 that can help you now:

- Treat yourself as a beginner.

- Focus on what you are trying to gain from the experience, not why you don't fit into the environment.

- Be open to a variety of different environments.

- Be an amazing planner.

- Introduce yourself to the instructor or fitness leader.

- If you know someone who is already in this community, go with them.

- It's ok to leave if it's just not right for you, but don't make this the norm.

- Work around your limits.

By keeping on top of these you'll be able to get the most out of the experience and be able to make the best decision on which fitness world will be best for you.

Like Baby Step 2 you can add one of these sessions into your three exercise sessions a week for the challenge in Baby Step 1 (which you will still be doing up until this point).

STRATEGY #2: Do a detailed assessment of each place you visit, both on a practical and emotional level

I love the idea of 'How does a musician listen to a song?'. Let me give you more detail here. If you are like me, when you find a song you love you end up playing it over and over again. Before I started playing the piano, if you asked me why I loved a certain song I probably would have used basic music language to explain why. Things like, 'I love the words', 'that guitar riff is cool', or 'she has a good voice'. I had a basic understanding of the song but I never thought about the musical choices the artists were making to create the thing I loved. This was because I was someone who enjoyed music—I was not a musician.

After learning the piano for a while I joined a band and we wrote and recorded some songs. One day I was having a piano lesson with my amazing tutor, Chris. I was kind of proud of one of our songs so I played it to him. Chris is an awesome musician, he's a man who has played at a very high level his whole adult life and would be in the top 5% of all people when it comes to music ability. When I played the song to him his comments weren't, 'I like that piano riff'. They were things like, 'I find it interesting how you dropped the third note from a major to a minor in the second bar of the riff'.

Chris was listening to music at a much deeper level than what most of us would. His observations dug into things like the choices we were making as a band and why we were doing this.

A higher level of observation is a great thing to have in Baby Step 3. Don't just understand how you feel, try to understand why the people in that environment make you feel that way and what they did to create this for you.

Here's a good example: I was recently coaching one of our sessions and a lady came along for the first time. At the end of the session she came up to me and said thank you for making her feel so welcome. This lady walked away from our session feeling welcomed, but what did I do to make her feel this way?

When she arrived I could see that she was new so I instantly went up to her and introduced myself, then I explained everything she needed to know about how the session would work. After that I introduced her to two of our runners who I knew would be of similar ability and asked them to share with her what it was like for them when they first joined the group. During the session I checked in on her often and made sure she had a clear understanding of the options she could use to make sure she was successful. Once we had finished I gave her a high five and a compliment on how well she had done.

There's a reason she felt welcomed. I had used a lot of basic techniques to create this for her and I cared about her feeling comfortable. When you experience the different environments in Baby Step 3 your aim is to tap into how you feel but also to understand what the people have done to create those feelings for you. This can be done on both what they did well and where they performed poorly. If you don't feel welcomed, why not? Use every experience to gain a deep understanding of what creates success.

With this in mind ask yourself these questions after each experience:

- What is the culture of this place?

- What were the top five feelings I had when I was there?

- What did they do to create these feelings?

- Do I feel this is an environment that will cater for my needs on this journey?

- Do they have a level that works for me?

Think about your answers to these questions after every experience you have.

STRATEGY #3: Ask other participants about the environment

This may be challenging for some people but there's real value if you can do it. While you are at each location, introduce yourself to another participant at the session. I can imagine that some people who are reading this may already be feeling some resistance. I get it. If you are new to exercise you may feel vulnerable in this early stage and want to keep to yourself but if you can make a small interaction you can gain some great insights about the environment.

One thing I've learnt about people is that they love to help others. I'm sure you are the same—when someone comes up to you and asks for help you are happy to help out. With this in mind a good strategy is to go up to someone, smile and say, 'Hi, I'm here for the first time and I would love to know if you have any tips for me in my first workout'. I can almost guarantee you will get a good response from people if you do this.

Once you have established this first interaction there's a question that can help you gain more insight: 'I'm thinking about joining this place, what would you say they do really well to help you with your fitness and where do you think they can improve?'. This is such a good tool because you will likely get an honest answer from someone who is an actual paying user. Most of your points of contact up until this point will be with people who are there to sell to you. They make their world look like it's the only answer for you and you only hear about the good stuff (which can be exaggerated), but if another participant tells you it's amazing, that has credibility.

The other benefit of this strategy is if you do determine that this is the world that you will commit to you would have already made your first connection!

If the environment has more of a one-on-one approach, like working with a personal trainer, it can be harder to do this. You can ask for testimonials but if they can't provide any this may be a good sign that they don't have much experience with beginners. Remember, you are looking for proof that they are a good fit for you.

STRATEGY #4: Go back to the ones that are appealing

After a few weeks you may find that you have one or two experiences that shine out from the others. At this stage go back and try those ones again. By now you'll have a good understanding of what feels good and it's worthwhile going back to see if it still feels good.

You don't want to have a 'fall in love with the first date' problem. You know the one—you go on a date with someone and it goes really well, you get all emotional, think this person is 'the one' and in your mind you build a picture of a future together. Then you have your second date and it's a disaster and you think, 'I'm glad I had this second date because this wasn't a good fit'.

Going back and experiencing the best options again will help to cement the best choice for you. You'll also see if they can consistently deliver a top notch experience.

STRATEGY #5: Determine which environment you will commit to

After four weeks of trying as many different providers of the movement you enjoy as you can, choose the one you will commit to. This is an exciting moment because the work you have done over the last few months has led to a point where you have found your exercise routine, the movement you enjoy doing, and now you are committing to your fitness world.

As you sign up for your new-found fitness community, be proud of yourself. You have done the work to get yourself to this place and it's exciting because your journey will actually get easier from here. Not so much on a physical level but more on a motivational and accountability level.

When you have a fitness community that you feel you belong to you want to turn up and it becomes an enjoyable part of your routine.

STRATEGY #6: Commit to being a part of this world

A few years ago I was taking the introduction seminar for Get up to Five. In the seminar I introduced the values of our business— growth, fun and community—and in the seminar there was a lady called Karin. You could tell that Karin was a shy type of person, she kept to herself, was more reserved in her nature, and she didn't answer any of the questions that I put to the group.

Karin's running story is an amazing one. She started with our beginner 5km group, when she was doing absolutely no exercise and went on to run 10km, a half marathon, and then a marathon. She's truly an inspirational example of how you can turn your exercise life around.

One Saturday morning after our run, the group was having coffee and I was having a chat with Karin. She said that when we had our introduction seminar for Get up to Five all those years ago and I talked about how community was an important part of what we do she thought to herself, 'That's not for me.' At that time she knew I could help her with running but she wasn't looking for a community and even resisted the idea of it because it wasn't her thing, but in the end the community was the biggest reason she achieved so much with her running and she learnt so much about herself by being a part of it.

I have a philosophy in life and it's really simple: 'I'm going to participate'. This means I'll sing a song at Karaoke even though I'm not the greatest singer. It means I'll introduce myself to someone in a new environment. It means I'll try new things. Ultimately 'I'm going to participate' means I'll embrace any opportunity that is put in front of me, even in areas I don't have a huge amount of confidence in.

Karin joined a world that had been designed to build community but for her to get the true value from this she had to embrace what that community had to offer. Even though this wasn't why she joined initially and it worked against her personality, she ended up embracing the community which has enabled her to achieve so much more than she ever thought possible and she now understands why this was so important to her success.

Once you have determined the community you are going to commit to, really commit to it. Start to make friends, embrace the things that your community does to create shared experiences and social bonding. Be a good presence in the community.

This may seem hard if you feel insecure and vulnerable around exercise or you may be a bit shy. Remind yourself that this community wants you to succeed and that the more you embrace it the more you'll have a group of people that you belong to. It's the community that will be one of the best parts of your exercise journey.

Mindsets to practise for Baby Step 3

- I'm aiming to get a deep understanding of what each option can provide for me.

- I'm going to be open-minded to every option available.

- I'm going to work through this process using all of the lessons I learnt in Baby Step 2.

- I will embrace each experience.

- I'm looking to find my community.

- Once I've found my community I'm going to participate in it.

Workbook for Baby Step 3

Baby Step 3, here we come. Again, we have a workbook for you to use throughout the next four weeks. This will help you get the most out of this Baby Step so by the end of it you will have found your community.

1. How do I make sure I keep the lessons from Baby Steps 1 and 2 in place throughout this week?

2. What are all of the options I can try around the movement I enjoy?

3. What option will I try this week?

Before you go to the first session:

1. What planning do I have to do to make sure I can have the best experience possible? (Getting there early, meeting the instructor, and knowing what gear I need).

2. How do I make sure I keep the lessons from Baby Step 2 in place during this experience? As a recap:

- Treat yourself as a beginner.

- Focus on what you are trying to gain from the experience, not why you don't fit into the environment.

- Be open to all of the different environments.

- Be an amazing planner.

- Introduce yourself to the instructor/fitness leader.

- If you know someone who already goes to this location, go with them.

- It's ok to leave if it's just not right for you, but don't make this the norm.

- Work around your limits.

During the experience:

How do I make sure I have a deep level understanding of the experience I am having when I'm there?

After the experience:

1. What did I like about the experience?

2. Were there things I didn't like?

3. Did I feel the leaders were able to help me on my journey?

4. Was there a community feel?

5. How did the community make me feel and do I feel this community could work for me?

6. Any other comments.

Repeat this process for all of your Weekly Meetings in this Baby Step.

Where to from here?

Baby Step 3 starts from here. Hopefully you are reading this towards the end of Baby Step 2 so in your next Weekly Meeting you'll do your planning around the different options for the movement you like.

By the end of the four weeks you should have your fitness world/community in place. This will be the one you continue on this journey with. In Week 3 come back and read the next step as you will need to do some planning.

Success in this step equals:

- You will maintain the lessons you've learnt in Baby Step 2.

- You will have tried all of the options available with the movements you like.

- You will have a deep understanding of what you need from your leaders and your fitness community.

- You will have found your fitness world and will be embracing and participating in it.

- You'll be ready to go onto the next Baby Step.

Imagine ...

If you had found a community in the movement you enjoy, a place where you felt welcome, supported and connected, imagine if you were surrounded by leaders and peers who understood how to guide and support you on your journey. By the end of this Baby Step this can be a reality. This is life changing stuff.

Share your Success

Once you have found your world go to our social pages and share it with us!
Use hashtag #myfitnessworld

To join our social pages go to:
www.passionaboutexercise.com/social

Remember you can sign up for the Passion for Exercise course by going to:
www.passionaboutexercise.com/course

Chapter 6

The number one key when setting your first fitness goal

I remember saying to my wife Jo, 'We have a problem'. It wasn't a relationship problem, it was a business problem. Get up to Five had been running for about four years and if you looked at our success rates, this programme was a total success. Nearly 90% of people who joined Get up to Five were successful in achieving the goal of running 5km in eight weeks with us. These people were unfit, often overweight and had given up on exercise. Most of our team continued on with their running journey with us and were creating massive change in their lives, both physically and mentally. We were so proud of what this programme was doing but our results weren't the problem.

The statistics from our marketing budget showed we got amazing results with our website hits and lead generation but they weren't transferring into sales. We were starting to hear the same comments from people who were joining the programme. They'd say that they'd looked at our website for over two years and had finally plucked up the courage to join.

The biggest problem was that the people we were trying to

help were afraid to join. The problem we had to solve was how to get people who want what we provide to actually do the thing they know will be good for them and commit to our programme.

Unfortunately, our solution was a total disaster but luckily there was a valuable lesson for us that came from it.

After sitting down and doing some thinking, we decided to create what we thought would be the perfect solution—we called it 'Stepping Up'. We thought that if beginner exercisers were so afraid of joining a beginner running programme we should start a four-week 'get ready to start running programme'.

The purpose of Stepping Up was to get beginners into the habit of exercising three times a week with a group. Within the sessions we had some beginner-level strength work and then the group would go for a walk. In the last week of the programme we would introduce some beginner running sets and by the end of the Stepping Up programme these people would feel more confident about moving up to Get up to Five.

For the next three months I worked my butt off creating Stepping Up and when it was ready to go I started the first marketing campaign. I was pretty excited because I felt we had the solution!

My excitement quickly deflated because we were making no sales. Nothing I was doing was working. As a business owner I've always tried to provide high-service products that have a higher price point because I feel you can do better work for your customers when you have this model. With Stepping Up it got to the point where I put it on one of those coupon sites, which is basically giving it away, and even then there weren't many sales.

In the end we did manage to get just enough people to run the first group but Stepping Up was a one-and-done product—we never ran it again. This was a very confusing time for us.

A few months later I was returning a phone call to someone who had left a message asking about Get up to Five; this was a sales call. During our conversation I was telling this lady about our success rate when she asked me why we thought we were so good at motivating people who have been unsuccessful with exercise. I gave the usual answers—the group dynamic, our coaching team, a wisely-designed programme—but then I said something I had never thought of before which kind of came out of nowhere.

'I think one of the keys to Get up to Five is that it gives beginner exercisers a goal that they really want to achieve. It's what I'll call a Proud Goal. We see it all of the time, when someone who hasn't exercised in years, is unfit and inactive goes on to run 5km, they are so proud of themselves. They put it on their social media feeds, they tell all of their friends about it, and they feel amazing about themselves.'

After I got off the phone I realised that I'd just had a lightbulb moment. The reason Stepping Up didn't work was because the goal we put in front of our people doing this programme wasn't a Proud Goal. 'Getting ready to run' isn't exciting, it's not sexy, you aren't going to put on your social media feed that you're ready to start running, you aren't going to feel super proud of yourself at the end of it.

Get up to Five was different; it was exciting and beginner exercisers would feel proud to tell their friends that they had run 5km. While beginner exercisers were fearful of Get up to Five, the goal was something that really appealed to them.

Unfortunately, when many people think about adding exercise into their life they have an 'I should' approach. They wake up one day feeling dissatisfied with their current health and fitness so they decide to make a change. This is an important moment but applying the 'I should' approach leads them to make choices that have good intent but lack what they really need to be successful. They join a gym because they feel they should exercise, they download some exercise app because they feel they should exercise, they plan to do some running because they feel they should. The problem with the 'I should' approach is, it's not very motivating or exciting.

There's a strategy in marketing called Future Pacing. This is where you communicate to your ideal customer in a way that makes them see themselves in the future with the result of what your product promises to deliver, and which shows them how their life will be better if they choose you. For example, when people join Get up to Five they see a future where they can run 5km and they imagine the benefits that will bring to their lives. This is exciting and it creates a desire which leads to motivation. This is what a Proud Goal does.

A Proud Goal has meaning, it gives you energy that you never knew you had before, it makes it attractive for you to grow as a person.

Obviously this Baby Step is going to be about you finding your Proud Goal but there's something just as important that sits alongside this.

Around two years ago Jo asked me if I could call a lady who had been emailing the business to get advice on how to train for a marathon. Jo told me that this lady wanted to do a marathon in five months from now but that she wasn't currently doing any running at all and didn't really have a running history. Jo had advised this lady that her plan wasn't a wise one but she wasn't getting through to her so we needed to give her a call to talk this through.

As soon as I started talking to this lady it became clear that she was very determined. She had decided that she wanted to do a marathon and there was no way I was going to talk her out of it. I was in a hard spot because she wanted us to guide her through this experience but I knew that her plan was unwise and would set her up for failure and possibly an injury.

After listening to her explain what she was aiming for I gave her my honest opinion that I wouldn't recommend she look to do this marathon within this very short time frame. It was way too ambitious for her current conditioning and her athletic history. I could tell that I wasn't giving her what she wanted to hear but I had to be honest. I advised her to give herself a year to 18 months to achieve the marathon goal and to start running with our 5km group and build up her running base in a wise and safe way.

Our conversation ended and it was clear that she was going to find someone else to help her with her marathon goal.

About six months later I received a phone call from the same lady. No surprises, she hadn't run her marathon. She hadn't even really started her training. She admitted that she'd struggled to even start running so her marathon goal had quickly been dismissed.

This was one of those times where honesty pays off. Because I'd been honest with her when we first talked she knew she could trust me and she ended up joining Get up to Five and did eventually run a marathon.

This is an example where a Proud Goal can go wrong. This lady's intent was amazing. She had found a goal that she would be proud of achieving, an achievement that would create an amazing future, but the problem was the goal was well above her current ability.

For a beginner exerciser you definitely need a Proud Goal but it's important you find one that is right for your current ability so you are setting yourself up for success. The goal can be a little bit scary and you know it will be a challenge but deep down you will believe you can achieve it. This is why our 5km programme is such a success, it's a Proud Goal that total beginners can safely achieve in the time frame we give them.

With all of this in mind here is Baby Step 4.

Baby Step 4: Find your Proud Goal that is set at the right level for your current ability

All the work you have done up until this point has been about getting you into your fitness habit, finding a movement you enjoy and finding your fitness community. Now you are ready to go on to the exciting stage in your journey—setting your first fitness goal.

This whole journey is about you growing as a person and getting to this point is proof that you have taken massive steps forward already. Now you are going to put specific energy towards achieving your first fitness goal. This is an exciting time and you will discover so much about yourself during this experience.

Challenge for Baby Step 4

Find your Proud Goal within the next two weeks that is set at the right level for your current ability.

The criteria to use for this is:

Would achieving this goal make me proud of myself?

I've already explained this so there's no need for more detail. Just think, 'Am I excited about achieving this goal? Would I want to tell my world about it?'

Is it realistic for my current ability?

You may not know the answer to this just yet. This is where your leaders and mentors are going to be really important. Have a chat to them about what you are aiming to achieve and whether or not you feel it's a wise option for you based on where you currently are within your fitness journey.

One thing that is really important here is that you must trust your fitness professionals. The story of the lady who wanted to run the marathon is a good example of this. Your leaders and mentors have a much better understanding of the safest and wisest pathway for your exercise progress. If they think you are aiming too high it can be disappointing but you have to trust them. If this happens, ask them what they feel would be a great Proud Goal for you right now and what are the stepping stones you need to take to get to your ultimate Proud Goal.

It might be that you would like to run a marathon so your stepping stone pathway will be to train to run 5km, then 10km and so on. Each stepping stone is a Proud Goal that is moving you towards your ultimate Proud Goal. Some exercise options already have this in place; think of the belt system in many martial arts or grades in local cycle racing.

The definition of current ability is broken down into physical and mental. With the physical, you are looking at your current physical condition and the skills you need to achieve your goal. With the mental, you are looking at the mind strategies you need to develop to overcome the mental hurdles you will face along the way. Again, this is why it is so important to have great leaders and mentors beside you. They will understand where you sit in both your physical and mental ability and they will be able to help guide you along the way.

By being successful in finding the right goal for your current ability you are giving yourself a much higher chance of finding a lifetime love of fitness. This is because you achieve the right level for your journey and will be learning and developing yourself, both physically and mentally, in the wisest way possible.

What if my movement doesn't have obvious goals?

There are some areas of fitness where the goals aren't so obvious. It may be that you have joined a gym and you love the classes but there's no clear goal that sits alongside these. If you are in this position look at the type of fitness goal the people who do these classes aim to achieve. It might be that you like a cycle class so you decided to sign up for your first ever entry level cycle race. You will find that if you spend some time digging into this there will be goals that people in your world work towards.

Rules for Baby Step 4

RULE #1: Trust the advice of your leader or mentor

At the risk of sounding like a broken record, but this is so important, setting your Proud Goal should be a collaborative experience. Use the wisdom of your leaders and mentors to your advantage and include them in your experience.

An important part of working with your leader and mentor is to trust their advice. I have this saying with some of my runners, it's 'Keenness is your enemy'.

I remember a really good example of this with one of our Get up to Five runners. This guy was in his late 50s and hadn't run in over 20 years. In designing our programme I've created a precise formula that safely conditions a person who has done no impact in a very long time. This plan needs to be precise because the risk of injury for an unconditioned person is high. The other thing that is really important in the early stage of their running journey is that they stay away from intensity. We advise our beginners to always run at or below 6/10 running where it feels easy and achievable.

At one of the sessions I was coaching I came up next to this guy and he was killing himself. The programme stated he was to do two minutes of light jogging followed by two minutes of easy walking. When I came up to him it was obvious that he was working too hard and I had my suspicions that he had gone longer than what the programme specified. So I asked him how long he'd been running for and he said he'd just hit ten minutes.

In a friendly way I advised him that he should stick to the programme and do the light jog/walk sets and he should pull back on the intensity. I told him that his risk of injury would go up massively if he didn't. He was a bit of a stubborn character because he told me he was feeling good and just wanted to see how he goes.

This man had paid for our service, had received the plan to follow which was proven to work, he was getting advice from someone who had trained thousands of people to achieve the goal he wanted to but his keenness had become his enemy. His 'I just want to see how I go' keenness was making him make foolish decisions.

The next week he had to withdraw from the programme because he got injured. This was such a shame because it didn't have to be this way. If he had trusted what we had created and taken the advice on board he would have been fine.

Keenness is an amazing thing, just don't let it lead to foolish decisions. Trust your leader and use their advice to help you make the best decisions.

RULE #2: The goal has to realistically fit into your life

'Keenness is your enemy' can also rear its head in this rule. You find a Proud Goal that you want to achieve and you get excited about achieving it but you don't realistically think about the practical obligation that comes with achieving this goal. This is one of the biggest mistakes new exercisers make.

I remember when I first started as a personal trainer I met with a client who wasn't doing any exercise when she came to see me. Before I could design her programme I needed to get an understanding of what she was hoping to achieve and what I needed to consider when putting her programme together.

When I asked how much time she had to train each week she told me that she could probably do 60–90mins a day. Alarm bells should have gone off in my head when she said this because up until this point in time she was doing zero exercise. In my lack of experience I didn't see this as a problem so I designed her a programme that required six days of training between 60 to 90 minutes each day.

Not surprisingly it was a total failure. After two weeks she had only done two sessions and this was my fault. If I was in the same situation today I would help this person figure out a more realistic level of exercise that could fit into her week based on the fact that she's a beginner and she is still learning how to add exercise into her weekly routine.

Up until now with the Baby Steps you have worked through, you will have discovered a realistic way of adding exercise into your life and at this stage in your journey, when you are thinking about finding a goal, use your current exercise schedule—or maybe just slightly more. Just don't add any more than what is realistic for you right now.

At the moment you might be doing three 30 to 45 minute sessions each week so setting a goal around the same type of schedule would be wise. You could add a little bit more, for example four sessions a week or extend the session times by 15 to 20 minutes and this would be the right amount of extension, but if you start to aim further than this you may be creating an unrealistic goal.

Again, work with your leaders here. They should have a good understanding of what it takes to achieve different levels of goals. Ask them if they think your goal is realistic around the time frames that work in and around your life.

Your Weekly Meeting will help as you have learnt more about your personal time management.

RULE #3: Involve your world and communicate with them about how they can help you

Ninety-nine percent of goals aren't achieved by one person alone—there are so many other people who help. For you to be successful you need to get your own world involved.

For example, if you are a parent with young children you may need your partner to be home at a certain time so you can get to your training session on time. Once you have your goal in place you want to communicate to your partner that on certain nights it's really important that they are home on time so you can get to your training.

Another example may be that you go to your boss and ask if you can start work 20 minutes later one day a week because you want to do a morning session. Let them know you are working towards this goal and it's important to you and you'd like a bit of flexibility with this start time one day each week.

By involving your world and communicating with them how they can help you, you are removing barriers that could make it harder for you to achieve your goal.

The examples I've shared are practical ones but you can also get your world to support you in other ways. Some things to consider are:

- How can people support you when you are lacking motivation?

- How can they help you feel good about what you are doing?

- What are other practical ways they can help?

There's another important benefit that comes with getting your world involved; the people that help you will feel a part of your experience and will want to lift you up along the way. You are building an amazing support team and they'll be with you right through to the moment you achieve your goal and they will be very proud of you when you do. They'll also feel some inner pride because of the support and help they have given you. Imagine if you had this support! What a great thing to have on your side!

With this in mind it's always important that you show your appreciation to your support team. Aim to show each of the people on your team how much you appreciate what they are doing for you.

Strategies to use in Baby Step 4

STRATEGY #1: Determine your goal

By following the Baby Steps and working with your leader, setting your goal won't be that hard because you have found the movement you enjoy and you are in a community of people who love this movement as well. We know you are just starting out with this and your community will have some clear beginner goals that you can work towards. Once you have worked with your leaders and mentors, set your goal in place with time frames around it.

That's right, you are now setting your first fitness goal.

This is such an exciting moment. You will now have a focus that you are moving towards. Be ready to grow.

STRATEGY #2: Have a goal setting session and create your plan

I had a cool experience last week. I was rummaging through some boxes in my garage when I saw a thick red bound book with the word 'Goals' written on it in my handwriting. I opened the book and saw that this was my first ever goals book from when I was 20 years old. This goals book was from before I even started working in the fitness industry.

For the next hour reading through it I was totally consumed. At that stage of my life I would redo my goals every four months and I was very thorough in that process. There were a series of questions I would ask and answer, assessments of where I was at in different areas of my life, and the actual goals and plans for each of the areas I wanted to work on.

One of the questions I would ask myself is, 'Where do I want to be in ten years from now?'. In one of the early goal-setting sessions in the book I had the answer: 'To be a world-leading fitness professional, to have financial freedom so I can choose to live my life how I want, to be able to live my life according to my values, and to be performing and writing music'.

It's been over 20 years since I wrote this answer down but today I am lucky to be a world recognised fitness leader, I'm financially free, I live my life to a higher level with my values and I'm playing in a band where we write and perform our own music. It's cool to think that what this 20-year-old version of me hoped for has actually come true.

The most important part to acknowledge is that this isn't a fluke. Living the life now that I wanted back then didn't come out of nowhere. It's something I've worked on and consciously created.

That's what setting goals does, they give us a focus and a plan. They point you towards where you are aiming to get to and design a plan for you to get you there.

The thing about a goal-setting session is that it takes effort and unfortunately for a lot of people their goal setting session is the thing they intend to do but never get around to doing. If you want to be successful on this journey this is such an important thing to do.

I have a strategy called 'How long is the actual cost of change?'. Let's say you have been using a piece of software for a few years and you are a bit of a guru with it, you know it inside out and know how to get the most out of it.

One day an email comes through from your manager about

upgrading the software. This email informs you that your job will be easier with the upgrade and how it will be better for your clients, plus it's inexpensive to get the upgrade.

The problem is, it looks a little bit different, the buttons aren't where they used to be and you may have to change some of your systems. You feel resistance, it seems like hard work and a lot of effort to make the change. What do a lot of people do in this situation? They don't do the upgrade—they stick with the familiar and don't change a thing.

A good question to ask yourself in this situation is, 'What is the actual time cost of me making the change?'. You may determine that it will cost you five focused hours of upgrading the software and then learning it. Then you ask yourself 'What are the benefits of me making this change?'. You determine that the upgraded software could save you two hours a week, would make your customer experience better, and would allow you to put your time into solving new problems.

As you can see, when you think of it this way, that five hours of effort becomes appealing. It seems like a small investment for a great return, which leads to you making the change.

Here are a couple of questions for you:

- How long will it take you to have a goal-setting session for the Proud Goal you have determined in this Baby Step?

- What will the benefits be if you have this goal setting session?

Based on my personal experience a goal-setting session for one area of my life takes under an hour to do and the benefits are huge. I have a better understanding of what it will take for me to achieve this goal and I have a plan in place on how to get there.

Be the person who puts the effort in, then you'll be the person who gets the benefits from this effort.

How do you set your goals?

There are a million books out there on goal setting. I'm a big believer that your goal setting process is something that evolves as you learn more and more about what works for you. In saying that, I want to share my process with you now.

Step 1:

My goal setting always starts with this question: 'Where am I currently in this area of my life?' Here, I give an honest assessment of my current position. This is important as it helps me to see where I can grow.

Step 2:

I determine the actual goal I want to achieve. A recent example of this is this book! At the beginning of this year I set the goal of getting this book written by the end of the year.

Step 3:

Before I get into the planning stage for my goal I like to explore obstacles or roadblocks that I may face along the way. This is really important because by identifying these now I can create a plan that I can implement if and when these roadblocks come up. Obstacles or roadblocks cover anything that will work against me achieving this goal. They can be practical things, personal character traits that work against me, or people who I feel will limit me.

Step 4:

I then form strategies for overcoming my obstacles/roadblocks. I'm looking for realistic and achievable strategies here. I try to ask myself, 'Is there a high chance this strategy will help me overcome this obstacle?'.

Step 5:

I identify the people who can help and how they can help me. Most goals need great people to help you along the way. Identifying them is key but also being clear on how they can help is just as important.

Step 6:

I create a plan to achieve the goal. This is where I get into the nuts and bolts of achieving the goal. I'm aiming to design a pathway to success. This is about identifying the actions I will take each step of the way. You may not have the exact steps set in stone by the end of this process but you will have a general idea of what you need to do to achieve the goal.

It's at this stage where you want to involve your leaders and mentors. They will provide you with the physical training plan that will wisely get you from where you are right now to a place where you are ready to achieve your goal. Their knowledge and experience is invaluable.

Step 7:

I use the 'I know I'm there when…' questions. This is about me having a clear picture of how I'll feel when I've achieved my goal and what that will look like.

Step 8:

What are the benefits of achieving this goal? Here's where I explore how my life will be better if I achieve this goal.

Step 9:

The last section is for any comments I want to note to myself.

As I said earlier, this is my process. You can give it a try or you may already have a goal setting process that works for you. My only comment would be, the most important thing is that you set your goal. Don't spend hours trying to find the right process. I'm sure 99.9% of goal-setting processes work, but only if you do them.

STRATEGY #3: Get feedback and make adjustments if needed

Once you have completed your goal-setting session it's a good idea to get your leaders and mentors to have a quick look over your plan, even the bits that aren't about the training. As they have been a part of your process already there probably won't be many changes that need to be made, but their experience and wisdom may be able to help find any adjustments that may need to be made. Take their advice on board and you'll have a better plan to help you move forward.

STRATEGY #4: Create a 'Goals Awareness' habit

Sitting down and writing your goals is a powerful tool in creating success but if you want to increase your chances of succeeding keep your goals at the forefront of your mind. This is where creating a 'goals awareness' habit is important as it will help you reflect on your goals throughout your week.

This doesn't have to be complicated. For example I have a quick scan over my goals every morning before I start my day, this only takes me two minutes. When my wife is training for a running race she will have her goals and her training plan on the fridge in our kitchen. Having her goals in a place that she sees each day helps remind her and keeps her awareness up.

What is the best way for you to put your goals awareness plan in place?

STRATEGY #5: Take a moment to be proud of yourself

Are you someone who knows you should do something but often doesn't end up doing it? If you are, you are not alone. Many people know they should exercise but they never do, they know they should plan their food but they never do, they know they should have that hard conversation with someone but they never do.

I find this dilemma an interesting one because the benefits of doing what you find hard to do are huge. If you exercise you are going to get healthier and fitter, you will feel great about yourself, you'll manage your weight better, and you'll be open to more life experiences. If you plan your food you'll eat the right portions of healthy foods, you'll save money because you eat less takeaway food, you'll eat less unhealthy food and you'll manage your weight better. If you have that hard conversation you remove the inner tension that avoiding the conversation brings, you'll deal with the problem you face, and if it's done in the right way you can create respect and a higher connection with that person.

We are so hard on ourselves when we don't do the things we know we should, and if we could just understand the benefits that would come from doing them, it's obvious! Goal setting is an obvious example, so many people know they should do it, they understand the benefits that would come but they still never do it.

By going on this journey you have joined the minority of people who actually do something they know will be good for them so it's important that you take a moment and pat yourself on the back. This isn't a small thing so don't diminish it. Take a moment to be proud of yourself for getting to this point and setting your goal.

Mindsets to practise for Baby Step 4

- I'm finding the right goal for my current ability.

- I want to find the goal that I'll be proud of achieving.

- I will use my leaders and mentors to help guide me towards the right goal.

- Goal setting isn't complicated or hard, I just need to do it.

- I will enjoy the goal-setting process.

- I'll feel proud of myself for completing my goal-setting process.

Workbook for Baby Step 4

This Baby Step shouldn't take a long time and it's important you plan the time needed during your Weekly Meeting. The longest you want to leave your goal-setting session is two weeks. Ideally you will get it done in a week. You could even aim to get it done within your next Weekly Meeting.

The Proud Goal I want to achieve is:

1. Where am I currently at in this area?

2. What do I want to achieve in this area?

3. What obstacles or roadblocks could I face in achieving this goal?

4. What strategies will I use to overcome these obstacles or roadblocks?

5. Who can help me achieve this goal and how can they help me?

6. How will I know when I have achieved this goal?

7. What are the benefits of me achieving this goal?

Create your plan/action steps that you will need to do to achieve your goal.

Any comments to add:

Once you have completed this process send it through to your leaders/mentors and if they offer suggestions, take them on board.

Where to from here?

Because Baby Step 4 should take no longer than a week or two you can continue onto Baby Step 5. While you are working through this process just keep your current exercise routine in place.

Success in this step equals:

- You will have the perfect Proud Goal in the movement you love, based on your current ability.

- You will have a plan in place to achieve this goal.

- Your leaders/mentors will have helped guide you in the process.

- You'll be excited to move towards the next Baby Step.

Imagine...

You have a goal that will make you feel super proud when you achieve it. By discovering this goal you feel a spark of energy that gives you the motivation to take yourself to a higher level. Imagine that you have a wise plan that your mentors have created for you and by following this plan you will achieve your goal. This is what you are heading towards now.

Share your Goal

Once you have found your Proud Goal go to our social pages and share it with us!
Use hashtag #myproudgoal

To join our social pages go to:
www.passionaboutexercise.com/social

Remember you can sign up for the Passion for Exercise course by going to:
www.passionaboutexercise.com/course

Chapter 7

What top athletes have taught me about goal attainment

I love reading books and watching documentaries about sports stars. I'm in my happy place when I'm learning about the lives of the athletes I have watched as a fan. That's why it's interesting that I somehow managed to miss the book and documentary about one of the greatest players in one of the sports I am most fascinated with in my own country—rugby.

In the game of rugby globally, there are just a handful of players that get mentioned when the 'greatest of all time' conversation comes up. But without fail, one name that comes up every single time is Richie McCaw. McCaw is a legend as both player and captain of one of the greatest sports teams in the history of this sport—the All Blacks.

McCaw played 148 games for the All Blacks in a career lasting 14 years which was made even more impressive because he played in one of the most physical positions in this very demanding sport. McCaw is the definition of success as a player. He won 88.5% of the games he played in and as a captain he had an 89.1% winning rate. He captained the All Blacks to two

World Cup wins—something no other international rugby captain has done—and won every trophy that a player could win in the sport. As much as I love rugby and was a total fan of this legend somehow I managed to miss his book and documentary when they came out.

One weekend I was travelling out of town to do a presentation at a fitness workshop. After a massive day of exercise I headed back to my hotel and as I was settling in for the night I turned on the TV. I was expecting to fall asleep within minutes because I was beyond tired. When I was flicking through the channels I saw that the Richie McCaw documentary was starting. I thought to myself, 'I'll give it ten minutes', knowing that my day would quickly catch up on me and I would probably be asleep in seconds.

Ten minutes went by and I wasn't asleep, I was wide awake and glued to the TV. I watched the whole documentary and I was 100% wrapped up in it. It had a lot of the traditional tropes of the usual documentary format—he'd overcome adversity to achieve the highest level in his sport—but the part I was most fascinated with was when Richie talked about setting goals and his approach to pressure moments during his career.

From an early age McCaw had always set high standards for himself, not just as an athlete but in all areas of his life. For this reason he achieved a lot but in his first period as the All Blacks captain the All Blacks lost at the World Cup, with arguably the best team at the tournament. This loss led to him exploring more of the mental side of being an athlete and captain.

The work he did during this time helped him focus on pressure. He explored the question of, 'How do you go from being a team that just survives under pressure to being a team that thrives?'. McCaw said that when you understand pressure you think, 'I need as much pressure as I can get because that's when you get good at it, so in the end the more pressure there is, the bigger the game, the better'.

Richie understands that he learns the most about himself when he has to face the high-pressure moments in his life. He puts himself in these high-pressure moments because he wants to be able to test and express himself at these times. To me, it seems like he loves achieving big goals but what he really loves is learning about himself and discovering who he is during his challenging moments. He also seems to enjoy discovering how he can navigate through these times in a successful way.

Richie McCaw is the elite of the elite so hearing him talk about facing a challenge can be a bit daunting. This guy has faced some of the biggest challenges possible in professional sport. When we think about where you are on your fitness journey there's no way I want you to be facing the level of challenge that Richie has, but there's an attitude that I want you to take with you on your journey that can be learnt from Richie.

In the last Baby Step you found your Proud Goal based on your current ability. You are now in the moment where you are going to start on the pathway of achieving your goal.

While getting the end result will be amazing and there will be so many benefits you will experience when you achieve it, I want to make sure you get the best value out of this time. That's why the next Baby Step isn't just 'Achieve your goal', it's...

Baby Step 5: Learn how to achieve your goal and enjoy the challenges along the way

When we set a goal we are aiming to be a higher version of ourselves. We want to be someone who can do something we aren't currently doing. In your goal-setting session you are creating a plan that will take you from where you are right now, to a place where you can do the thing you want to do. These plans are important—they give you a pathway to follow as you move towards achievement—but the real hurdles are faced when you start moving down that pathway. Being a goal setter is a great thing, most people don't get this far, but being a *goal achiever* is the next level.

This Baby Step is about you achieving your first fitness goal but more importantly it's about learning how you achieve goals and approach them them with an attitude of excitement by the challenges you will face. This is where you can be like Richie.

Challenge for Baby Step 5

This one is pretty simple: you are now aiming to achieve your goal. In doing this you are looking to have the approach of 'I'm learning how to achieve a goal and I'm going to face and enjoy the challenges along the way'. Exciting times.

Rules for Baby Step 5

RULE #1: Only focus on the achievement of this goal

In Baby Step 4 we spent time helping you find the right goal, your Proud Goal that is set at the right level for your current ability. You should now have this in place.

One of the biggest hurdles people face in goal achievement is the loss of focus. There can be many reasons for this, one of these being that *you need to achieve more than the goal you are aiming to achieve.* This reminds me of a lesson I learnt when I was about six or seven years old.

When I was younger my father had a drinking problem; he was an alcoholic. It was an addiction that caused many problems throughout his life and he got to the point where he decided he needed to give up drinking for good. Wisely, he went through a treatment programme to support him through this challenging change but drinking wasn't my dad's only vice; he was a big smoker as well, smoking a packet a day. For my dad's long-term health, giving up the drink was important but giving up smoking was needed as well.

It's funny what you remember because I was only young when he was going through this but I clearly remember having an interaction with my dad that taught me an important life lesson.

From what I remember my Mum had given up smoking before my dad went into his treatment programme so I understood that smoking wasn't good for you. One day I was talking to dad and

I asked him if he would be giving up both smoking and drinking at the same time. He told me that the people who were helping him told him to not worry about stopping smoking while he was working on giving up drinking. They had told him to put all his focus on winning the alcohol battle and once he had done that he could then put his energy into stopping smoking.

Something must have clicked inside my young head because I remember thinking that that made complete sense. I'm really proud of my dad because he gave up drinking completely at that time and not long afterwards he gave up smoking as well. These are two of the hardest habits to break and he overcame both of them. His success was helped because he focused on changing one of these at a time.

Change like this is helped when you have great mentors around you that you listen to. It's a lesson that you need to remember at this stage of your journey.

Often when people have put goals in place they get distracted, and often it's because they start setting more goals along the way. They may set a fitness goal, but then they also set a weight loss goal, a learning goal, and a relationship goal. While the intention is coming from the right place, when they set more goals the approach leads to failure because they overload themselves and put an unrealistic load in place.

A lady I know who's a leading development psychologist for high-level business leaders always reinforces to me that you should only ever focus on changing one or at maximum two things at a time.

While you may want to lose weight, learn a new language, and develop your relationship skills, adding them on top of this journey will only work against you. Be like my father, just focus on the achievement of this one goal.

Another reason people lose focus is that they look ahead of their current level and want to achieve that level when they aren't ready. The sport of triathlon shares a good example of this. Triathlon has different versions of its races. There's a sprint race, which takes between 50-70 minutes, the Olympic distance which is between 2-3.5 hours, the 70.3 distance which is between 4-8 hours, and lastly the Ironman which is between 8-17 hours.

All of these different distances have their appeal but the one that is the ultimate golden ticket for many triathletes is the Ironman. You may have seen an Ironman race or at least a promotional video or news clip. They are appealing to watch because they show every day people achieve amazing things and this makes people believe that they can do this too. It's powerful stuff.

Often people get into the sport of triathlon by starting at sprint race level—the perfect level for a beginner. While they are going through this journey in their head they are thinking about doing an Ironman triathlon—they are attracted to the golden ticket of the Ironman. Having ambition is a good thing but if this ambition takes the focus off your current goal it is ultimately taking you off your path.

One of my good mates, and world-leading triathlon coach, John Newsom has what he calls 'The John Newsom three year plan'. This is a plan that takes a total beginner from doing nothing to doing an Ironman. With John's plan you'll do a few sprint distance triathlons, then some Olympic distance races, then a couple of 70.3s, and then you are ready to face your first Ironman challenge.

In each step of John's plan you use the different levels of triathlon racing to help you learn the right lessons at the right time so that when you sign up for your first Ironman you are 100% prepared, both physically and mentally.

So, if you find yourself looking ahead of your current goal at this stage of your journey, enjoy the fact this is happening but stop yourself from allowing this to distract you from the lessons you need to learn at this stage of your development.

Keeping focused on only achieving this goal is a good approach to have, it will allow you to put all of your energy into the aspects that will create success for you. So if you catch yourself adding more goals or looking ahead of the goal you have set for yourself, remind yourself that this is working against you.

RULE #2: Be process focused

It's been interesting watching interviews with sports people over the last few years whether it be individual athletes or a team. No matter what the sport is, it's like there is a universal language that they all seem to share when they talk about what they are focusing on. It's 'process-driven' language. You may already be aware of this. If not, next time you are watching an interview see if you can hear these people talk about this—their process to achieve success.

So what is process-driven focus all about?

When most of us think about goal setting we think about the outcome. It might be to run 5km, to do a bodybuilding competition, to achieve a certain result with a sports team. This outcome often has many benefits attached to it, for example you might think, 'If I run 5km I'll be leaner and fitter and my friends will be impressed with me'.

Having a desired outcome is a good thing because it gives you a vision of what you could be, but as soon as you start taking actions towards achieving your goals you want to shift your focus away from the *outcome* and instead focus on the *processes* you need to implement to give yourself the highest chance of success in achieving your goal.

Let's break this down. Let's say you have the outcome goal of running 5km—a Proud Goal you want to achieve—and you feel your life would be better if you could do this. Now that you have this goal in place, what are the things you actually need to do to achieve this? The list would include things like:

- Get a programme that will work for your level of ability.

- Plan your training in and around your life and other commitments.

- Learn how to manage the running journey.

- Develop motivational tools to help.

Once you have your overall plan in place, break down each step into processes. This could be something as simple as, 'What is the process I need to make sure I get out the door today to do my training?'.

The process you need to focus on may include:

- I need to pack my bags before I go to work.

- I need my partner to look after the kids when I get home.

- I will drive straight to the park as soon as I finish work.

- When I start my run I will focus on easy running and I will listen to my breathing to make sure I'm not breathing too hard.

- At the halfway point I will put my most motivational workout music on and practise using positive affirmations that put my focus on the right area.

- In the last part of the run I will focus on the technique advice my coach has given me.

You can see that if you focus on the process rather than the end goal, there's a much higher chance that you will not only do your run, you will do it in a successful manner. You are building towards your ultimate outcome, one process at a time.

I'll give you another quick example. If I want to get some productive work done (the outcome I desire) my process is:

- I plan time in my diary when this work will be done.

- In the morning I do some visualisation around doing this work.

- I plan this work after a break in my day, because I know I'll have better energy both physically and mentally.

- Before I start, I get a piece of paper and write down the objectives I want to achieve which are clear and realistic based on the time frame I have set.

- I remove all distractions before I start the work.

You can see that by putting my focus on the above process there's a huge chance that I will get this work done to a high level, which was the initial outcome I wanted.

So, as you face each step in your challenge use these questions:

1. What is it I want to achieve today?

2. What is the process I need to focus on to help me achieve this?

3. How can I increase the chances of me taking the actions in my process?

Then put all of your focus into working through these process steps.

I don't expect you to be a rock star with this straight away but if you put this thinking in place and learn what works best for you, you will continuously take the actions needed which will lead to you achieving your goal.

Strategies to use in Baby Step 5

STRATEGY #1: Use your 'Success Formula'

In my first book I introduced the concept of a Success Formula. If we go back to Richie McCaw, he was a hugely successful rugby player but his success didn't finish there. He's gone on to do extremely hard endurance sporting events, has become a pilot, and has very successful business ventures. Richie McCaw isn't just a successful rugby player, he's a successful person.

It seems that Richie takes the lessons he has learnt from success in one area of his life and then applies them into his new endeavours. The more challenges he faces the more he knows how to be successful. This is what I call your Success Formula.

The Success Formula starts with the understanding that you have been successful in something in your life. Before we do this, let's look at how we define success. A good way to think about where you have been successful is to look at situations where you have put a conscious effort into improving an area of your life.

If you think about this now, you will be able to find areas where you have had success based on this definition. It might be that you wanted to learn how to cook a new meal, it could be an education achievement, up-skilling in your career, or a hobby like playing a song on a guitar. Right now, identify one area that you have been successful in.

Now reflect on the strategies you used to achieve it. What tools and strategies helped you? Try to dig deep here, don't just say 'I made it a priority', say 'I planned my weeks to make sure I had the time and focus to do the study that I needed to do'. The deeper you dig the greater insight you will gain.

Once you have reflected on this area, look at another area where you have experienced success. Again, what tools and strategies did you use? Ideally you want to write down all the different tools and strategies that you have used during your successful times.

At the end of this process you will have a list of tools and strategies that have worked for you in the past. This is your Success Formula.

So what are you going to do with this? It's simple; you are aiming to apply these tools and strategies to the goal you are aiming to achieve right now.

Spend some time looking at the tools and strategies from your Success Formula and ask yourself how they can help you be successful on this current journey. Then set in motion how you are going to apply these.

The great thing about your Success Formula is that it can always be evolving. Achieving your current fitness goal is going to teach you more about how to be successful, which you can apply as you move forward in life.

STRATEGY #2: Have a 'Bad Day Plan'

In Baby Step 1 Strategy #7 was 'When you have bad days, don't make them bigger than what they are'. This is a strategy that is important for this Baby Step as well.

Let's get this out of the way right now—you are going to have bad days. There may even be times where you have a few bad days in a row. This will suck, you will feel unmotivated, doubt will probably fill your head, and giving up may seem appealing. The first thing to recognise is that this is all part of the journey and that it's your job to keep turning up the next time. This understanding helps but we also want to be prepared for these times.

The best way to do this is for you to have a Bad Day Plan. This is a plan that you will use to make sure you do the next session. This plan is a little more involved than the one I gave in Baby Step 1, because you are now in the day-to-day goal achievement stage.

Here are some things to include in your Bad Day Plan:

- Acknowledgement: This is important; accept it's a bad day but don't let it build into a story. The bad day doesn't have to represent anything bigger, it's just a bad day.

- Have a learning approach: Explore why you had a bad day and see if there are some learnings in there for you. Sometimes you just have a bad day but other times you can see how you worked against yourself. It might be that you stayed up too late watching TV so you were tired before a key session. This will teach you to get to bed earlier before key training days.

- Put your focus on the next session and make it as appealing as possible: The most important thing to do after a bad day is turn up and do the next session. If you miss the next session and this continues for a few times you can fall off your goal wagon. So once you get in from your bad day, put all of your energy into making sure you do the next session. You want to make it as easy as possible mentally to do the next session. Tell yourself that you can go as easy as you want with the intensity of the next session. You may plan to meet up with a friend or you let your coach know that you need to be let off the hook for the next session.

- Remind yourself of the good times: Often when we have bad days we can get forgetful. We forget that we have had many enjoyable moments on our journey, because we can be emotionally struggling and our focus concentrates on why everything is so hard. This emotionally-driven negative place often isn't reflective of the real experience you have been having, it's one moment. Spend some time looking back over what you have been doing and see the moments you have enjoyed, making sure you see them in all the different areas that are a part of this journey. You can look back and see when you had fun with your training group, when you had a breakthrough moment with your skill development, when you felt good about yourself because of the intensity you hit. It could be as simple as seeing something that was beautiful in nature. When you are in the 'this sucks' place, try and look back and see all the positive experiences. It allows you to keep things in perspective and makes it easier for you to turn up the next time.

- Prepare a Personal Motivation Statement: A couple of years ago I got a text on a Friday night, the night before one of our 5km final run days. It was from one of our runners who was aiming to run 5km for the first time. This person had let me know that she had suffered confidence issues over the years. She texted to say that she wouldn't be there in the morning, she just didn't think she could do it.

As a coach I 100% believed she could run 5km. Over the last eight weeks she had turned up to every session and done the training required to run 5km. She was 100% physically able to do this but this moment of doubt led to her wanting to quit.

I knew she wanted support from me at this moment and that she didn't want to quit, it just seemed overwhelming. I gave her a call and talked through the reasons why I believed in her. I lessened the expectations by telling her she can turn up and walk the whole thing, but I also told her to go back and read her Personal Motivation Statement. In our introduction seminar we get our runners to write down their Personal Motivation Statement and I tell them to use this tool when they are struggling so that they continue on their journey.

The next morning she didn't just turn up, she ran 5km nonstop for the first time in her life—it was pretty cool. After her run I asked her what helped her overcome the barrier she had faced the night before. She told me that she had gone back and read her Personal Motivation Statement, which stated, 'I will always turn up, no matter what'.

In this most challenging mental moment, going back and reading her Personal Motivation Statement allowed her to overcome a place where she was going to quit. This is a great tool to have on your side.

The key thing with a Personal Motivation Statement is that you have it written down and that it's easily accessible. As a part of your Weekly Meeting this week you could include time to write down your Personal Motivation Statement.

- Learn what works for you. As I was saying earlier, you are going to have bad days. I've offered some strategies that can help but learn what will work for you. This is why bad days aren't a bad thing, they are just a learning opportunity. While you will never remove the bad days, how you respond to them can massively shift you so you can get to a place where they never take you away from your path.

STRATEGY #3: Build evidence of positive exercise experiences

Have you heard about the Fitness Fortune Teller? Trust me, they are terrible at their job.

A fortune teller's job is to tell you what your future will look like; you may or may not believe in the idea of a fortune teller but if indeed there was an amazing one nearby, they would be able to paint a clear picture of what your future looks like.

We all have our own Fitness Fortune Teller which gives us the perspective of what our future exercise experience is going to be like and the reason most people's inner Fitness Fortune Teller is so terrible at its job is that they predict that exercise is going to be hard, that it's going to hurt, that you will quit, and that there will be no enjoyment.

Let's take a step back—if you feel something is going to be hard, that it's going to hurt, that you won't enjoy it and that you will quit, how appealing will that thing be? Not at all!

If you put the right steps in place, like finding the right level of exercise for your conditioning, exercise often delivers the best feelings and experiences in your day. Sure, we have the odd bad day but the majority of the time exercising is an overwhelmingly positive experience. You feel good about yourself, you make physical changes, you overcome challenges, often you have fun social interactions, you can get to enjoy nature... the list goes on and on.

The bit I find fascinating is that people can experience these amazing positive benefits but still look at the next session with the Fitness Fortune Teller's perspective—that it's going to be hard, it will hurt, and so on.

We need to get good at building evidence that disproves our Fitness Fortune Teller. This is about seeing and attaching the good experiences to your inner perspective. The best way to do this is after you have finished every session reflect back on what value it brought to your life, looking at all the different aspects that session delivered. You could identify that it was a great stress release from your day, that you enjoyed the interaction you had with other people, that you felt great about yourself at the end of the session. Again, the list goes on.

As you build evidence of your positive fitness experiences, the way you look at your future sessions will shift. You'll understand that they will bring a lot of good to your day, so instead of wanting to stay away from them you will want to move towards them because your evidence proves your life is better with exercise in it.

A simple way to approach this is to give yourself a few moments to reflect as you leave your fitness session. Ask yourself how you feel, what you enjoyed, why this was good for you, and then remind yourself of these things when you think about doing the next session.

One thing you will often hear me say is, 'People who are successful with health and fitness are people who prioritise it'. One thing that nearly all of these people have in common is that they understand that their life is better because they exercise. By getting good at seeing how much value exercise brings you in all areas, the more you will become one of the people who prioritises it.

STRATEGY #4: Use your support network

We have spent a bit of time on this already so just to reiterate, when you are in goal achievement mode your support network is very important. Use them to guide and support you as much as you can. These people are a big part of your success, use them to your advantage. The key things to reinforce about your support network are:

1. Stick to the plan from your mentors/coaches.

2. Communicate clearly how they can support you in achieving this goal.

3. Show gratitude towards their support.

STRATEGY #5: Have a challenge/growth mindset

Many of you will know about fixed vs growth mindsets. The concept was introduced by Psychologist Dr. Carol Dweck and it has had a huge influence in many fields.

The basic way to look at this is that the two different mindsets massively affect how you approach things. When you have a fixed mindset you have an 'I can't grow in this area' approach. It's interesting because people often reveal the areas they are fixed in by saying things like 'I can't play music', 'I can't run', or 'I'm not creative'. You may have made some similar comments yourself.

The problem with fixed mindsets is that because you feel you can't do a certain thing, you don't even bother giving it a try. If you can't play music, why would you pick up a guitar? If you can't run, why would you bother downloading a 5km app? When you are fixed in your mindset you aren't even willing to open the door to trying. Ironically this just reinforces your fixed mindset because you will never build experience to disprove your inner thinking.

Then we have a growth mindset. This is when you understand that you have the ability to grow in any area of your life. Instead of thinking, 'I can't play music' you think 'If I'm willing to put time and effort into playing the guitar I know I can improve'. You can see how this different inner framing leads you down a completely different path, one which allows you to grow.

Obviously I want you to have a growth mindset in this journey but I want to share a tool that I introduced to my clients which helped people apply the growth mindset much more effectively. I call it Bevan's Growth Grading System.

When I first started introducing the fixed vs growth concept to my clients I discovered that there was a big problem. My clients understood that having a growth mindset was wise but they often got lost on where to aim their growth, and often when they did set a goal for growth, they set it too high. Here's an example:

I was never a good place-kicker of a rugby ball. If a game of rugby was dependent on me kicking the winning points, you would definitely bet your house on me missing (and you would make a lot of money). I'll admit that I had a fixed mindset of 'I can't place-kick'. Now let's say I decided that I wanted to improve my kicking and I shifted my thinking from 'I can't place-kick a rugby ball' to the growth mindset of 'I know that if I put in time and energy and get good advice I can definitely get better'. This growth mindset has opened me up to doing the work to get better but at the same time I have a problem, where do I start?

This problem often leads to people quitting because the starting point is too high. In my example I might watch some online videos that teach kicking skills but they are targeted at already competent kickers so when I go and practise I get confused and end up feeling like I'm failing. Unfortunately this experience reinforces the fixed mindset of 'I can't kick'.

With this in mind a better way to approach the challenge of 'Where do I start?' is to use Bevan's Growth Grading System (by the way, I made that name up for this book).

After I have shifted my mindset to growth, the next thing I do is ask myself on a scale of 1-10 where do I sit with my place-kicking ability and skill?

At this point in time you are aiming to accurately assess your current ability based on your skills, both physically and mentally, and grade yourself accordingly.

With me, I would give myself a 1/10. The reason is I don't miss the ball when I kick it but I have no understanding of where to look, what type of run up I should have, where I should aim to connect my foot with the ball when I kick, I don't know what to think when I'm kicking, and I don't know how to consistently get the height and distance needed. I'll be honest there's probably a lot more to add to this but you get the idea.

Now that I have an understanding of my current skill level, the next thing is to determine the different skills required at each level. Let's say they look something like this (again I'm no kicking expert):

0 – You miss the ball completely.

1 – You are able to connect your foot with the ball.

2 – You know where to look when you are kicking the ball.

3 – You have your run set in motion.

4 – You know where your foot should hit the ball.

5 – You know what should be happening with your body when you kick the ball.

6 – You have an understanding of how much weight to put on the ball when you kick it.

7 – You know what to think about when you go through the whole process.

8 – You are able to account for external factors like the wind or rain.

9 – You do all of the other skills consistently.

10 –You are able to calm your mind and 100% deliver when the pressure is at its highest.

Because I have done my personal skill assessment, where I gave myself a 1/10, and I have gained an understanding of the skill development pathway (which I would recommend that you do with a wise mentor), which has the scale of 1-10, I now know where to start. Based on the above scale I would start my kicking growth pathway by becoming competent at level 2, which is understanding where to look when I'm kicking the ball.

What I like about this approach is that it allows you to shift your inner dialogue and refine your growth mindset statement. Instead of saying, 'I know that if I put time and energy and get good advice I can definitely get better' I can frame it like this: 'Currently I'm a grade 1 kicker and I know that by putting in time and effort and getting good mentoring I can develop my ability to get to grade 2'.

As you read this you can see that my growth seems so much more achievable. First, there's the shift in mindset from fixed to growth, and second, there's a growth pathway that allows me to see where I need to put my focus and energy. Once I get to grade 2 of my goal kicking journey I can redefine my growth statement and also tweak my pathways so now I'm focusing on the skills of level 3.

With all of this in mind give yourself time to develop your growth statements and your development pathway. With your growth statements you could come up with an overall statement, like 'I know that by putting the effort in and getting great advice I will grow as a basketball player', and then you could refine further in areas where you know you are fixed in your thinking, like 'My free-throw will improve by me practising pointing my elbow towards the hoop when I shoot'.

With your skills, think about Bevan's Growth Grading System. Use your mentors to gain a greater understanding of where your current skills are and where the next level is. This will allow you to be able to put your focus on what is important.

Once you have done this work, note when you are going back to thinking habits that work against you. If you catch your inner dialogue having a fixed focus, redirect your thinking back to your growth mindset. If you are trying to develop skills that you aren't ready for yet, remind yourself that this is a skill building process and that you are best to focus on your current level.

STRATEGY #6: Evolve your ability to get feedback

When I first started teaching group fitness I had a burning desire to become one of the best in the world and there was no stone that I was going to leave unturned to achieve this. I did everything, and I mean everything, to be the best that I could be. I was so determined to achieve this level that I even had affirmations that I would read every morning that were focused on becoming the best. Some would say I was a bit over the top.

I'm proud to say that ultimately this time led to me achieving my goal of being a world leading fitness professional. Looking back there were many things that led to my success but one of the most important factors was my seeking of feedback and my ability to take it on board.

When I think back on how I used feedback there were different ways I applied it. They included:

- **Self Assessment:** I would film myself teaching every week and watch it to see where I could improve.

- **Member feedback:** This was from the members who did my classes. Their feedback helped me understand what they enjoyed about my experience and where they felt I could improve. They would share with me what the greatest instructors did, which gave me valuable insight into where I should aim to grow.

- **Peer feedback:** This was feedback from people of the same level as me. We would help each other by being honest about our abilities.

- **Leader feedback:** Managers and high-end trainers who had higher level knowledge and insight which revealed things I couldn't understand at that stage in my development.

- **Guru feedback:** I actually sent a video of my teaching to one of the best instructors in the world and they kindly sent me back in-depth feedback that was of the highest level.

Getting feedback is one of the best ways to improve and it's important that you have different ways of getting that feedback, but more importantly, your ability to take on and apply the feedback is the real key to your success.

I've been fortunate to be a leader of others in my life. I've had a lot of experience in giving feedback to others and I've learnt that there are different types of people when it comes to receiving feedback. Some examples include:

- The 'Sponge': This person is the best person when it comes to feedback. They love receiving it, they understand what the feedback is and where they need to put their energy and focus as they progress forward.

- The 'Defender': This person isn't able to take on feedback because they aren't open to listening to what is offered. They will come back with reasons why the feedback is wrong or reply with justifications of why the current experience isn't typical so the feedback doesn't really count.

- The 'You Just Don't Like Me': This person takes the feedback as a personal attack or as an emotional beat up. They feel the person giving them feedback is being unfair because they dislike them.

- The 'Can See Through My Insecurities': This person feels like everyone can see their insecurities so when they get feedback they feel that this has worked against them.

- The 'I don't understand': This person is willing to take on feedback but they don't gain the right understanding of where they need to improve, so once the feedback has been given they can apply their energy to the wrong areas.

There are plenty of other examples of how people deal with feedback. For you to be successful in this Baby Step you need to learn how you deal with it and aim to become a Sponge with your feedback.

Spend some time gaining an understanding of how you currently deal with feedback. If you discover that you are restricting yourself you could practise this easy five-step method:

The 'Getting the Most from your Feedback' method

1. Before the session, be aware of how you could potentially reject feedback. This is about you knowing how you could work against the process and having the ability to stop yourself when you catch yourself doing it.

2. Remind yourself that the person giving you feedback

wants to help you. As long as you have chosen the right person on your team they will want to help nurture your growth, so before you get feedback remind yourself that they are coming from a place of wanting to help you grow.

3. Listen and try to understand the learning when you are getting feedback. Getting feedback can be an ego-driven experience and you can have emotional hits and rewards. While this will probably always have a place within feedback we want to shift away from it being an ego experience to being one where our focus is on being curious. Ultimately we want to be in a place where we are trying to get as much understanding of the feedback we are receiving as possible. To help with this, think to yourself 'I'm a reporter who is aiming to gain the greatest understanding from this person by listening and using good questions'.

4. Show understanding: Once the person has given you the feedback, communicate back to them what you have understood. This helps create alignment and if there has been a misunderstanding it can be sorted.

5. Create a plan: With both of you knowing you are on the same page you can develop a plan of how you will progress in the area you have been given feedback in.

This method allows you to get out of your own head and gain the understanding, and the planning, that will help you move forward. By doing this you will fast-forward your progress because that's the true value of feedback.

Ideally you should be aiming to be getting a lot of feedback during this Baby Step. I guarantee that if you do, you will massively increase your chances of success, but it also gives you an ability to get better at using feedback in all areas of your life. It's such a powerful tool to have when you are growing so embrace it and make the most of it.

STRATEGY #7: Good on top of good, on top of good

Do you know what I love? I love running. There's something about this movement that takes me to a place where my mind gets to drift away. When I'm in this place I solve all my problems and can think about my future with ambition and excitement.

Do you know what I love even more than running? Running whilst listening to my favourite music. I have a music playlist that I call 'fast running'. Every song in this playlist is a song I absolutely love. When one song finishes and the next one starts playing I think to myself, 'I love this song!'. When I'm running with music it triggers emotional states that are so rewarding for me.

Do you know what I love even more than running with music? Running with music in beautiful nature. There's something about running on a hilly trail or in a forest that makes me feel aligned as a person. I believe all humans need time with nature so when I combine running, music and nature I feel a sense of oneness with myself and the world. I always have this inner thought that I'm making great decisions in my life when I'm in this place.

Do you know what I love even more than running with music in beautiful nature? Running hard with music in beautiful nature. I love intense running, that place where your body is moving fast and there's an inner challenge but because you are fit you know you can stay in this place. There's a reward that comes with this that's hard to describe. When I'm running fast with music in beautiful nature I'm in my most satisfied place, it's almost the best of what life has to offer.

What I have described is what I call the Good On Top Of Good strategy. As a part of your goal achievement there are many different actions and activities that you are going to have to do. There's training, then planning, the feedback sessions, the skill development, and so on. In a perfect world you would love doing every part of them but we all know that that's highly unlikely. There will be some activities that you love doing and some that you avoid doing. This is where the Good On Top Of Good strategy comes into play.

Let's break it down in two different ways: the activities you enjoy and those you struggle with.

With the activities you enjoy, look for deeper ways to make them appealing. My running example shows this. I already love running so it's easy for me to get out the door and go for a run but when I think about running fast in nature with music I experience a higher level of motivation. Then I'm excited to have my running time because I know it's going to be a highlight of my day.

With the activities that you enjoy in your goal journey, how can you make them Good On Top Of Good? What parts can you add to make it even more attractive for you to do that activity?

Then we have the activities that we struggle to do. When you think about doing them it's not appealing at all and you find yourself looking to avoid them. It's these activities that you feel you need to really motivate yourself to do.

Let's say your goal at this stage in your journey is to complete a 40km local bike race with a couple of hills in it. You find that you are good at getting out and doing your training except you struggle to do the hill repeat sessions that your coach has put in your programme (in case you don't know what hill repeats are, it's where you ride up and down a hill continuously for a set period of time).

Whenever you think about doing this session you start talking yourself out of it, you only see that it's going to be hard so it's not appealing at all. At the same time you know you need to get it done to be successful in achieving your cycling goal. This is a good time to put the Good On Top Of Good strategy in place.

What you know about yourself is that you love a beautiful view so you choose a hill that has the most amazing view so every time you reach the top you get a visual reward. You also know that you are more motivated when you are training with others so you plan a group hill repeats session every week (which also has a coffee catch up at the end of it). You make an 'I'm a badass hill climber' playlist which has the most motivational songs in it. Lastly you buy yourself a hill climber's cycle top, it's the one that your favourite cyclist wears. You only put this top on when you do your hill repeats and when you put it on you feel your inner super human come out.

Using the above example—riding with motivating music, on a course that has a visual reward, with a group of cycling friends, in your superhuman top—makes it attractive for you to do the session that you would normally avoid.

Have fun with the Good On Top Of Good strategy but more importantly put it in place where you know there are aspects to your journey that you are shying away from. You may find that if you use this strategy wisely those sessions you want to avoid actually become your favourite.

This also counts for the parts of this journey that aren't physical training. It could be doing the event planning, mental skills training, or your performance plan. Many people will neglect some of the other things you need for success. If you find you are doing this, remind yourself to use the Good On Top Of Good strategy.

STRATEGY #8: Your performance day is a learning experience

We all want to have that amazing experience of achieving a massive goal. It's that moment where you cross the finish line of something you have worked hard to achieve, where you get overwhelmed with emotion because this means so much to you. These moments make the hard work all worth it.

I want you to have an experience like this and if you have chosen a wise first goal based on your current ability and have stuck to your plan, there is a high chance of you experiencing this. Sitting alongside this you also want to learn about performing on your day.

In my time as an Ironman there were many athletes to be impressed with. There were the everyday people achieving their first Ironman triathlons right up to the world-class athletes who were aiming to win the race. I admired all of these people because in my mind they were all putting themselves in a challenging situation where they were testing themselves, and ultimately learning about themselves. While I had admiration for everyone within a race, the athletes I admired the most were the world-class athletes who consistently delivered to their highest level in every race.

I did Ironman for six years and in that time there were probably four or five professional athletes who delivered this high standard. They didn't just have some great races in a year, they delivered in every race. I'm sure you can think of athletes in sports that you love that live up to this standard. It's those athletes who always seem to deliver no matter how hard the challenge is.

People of this level have many things going for them, one of them being that they have figured out how to perform in their time of challenge. This isn't something they are born with, it's something they have learnt and they have learnt it by building up experiences of challenging moments and then learnt all of the parts of the puzzle that creates an amazing performance.

I want your performance day to be a rewarding one that delivers on the highest emotional level but I also want you to treat it as a learning experience. If the goal of this book is for you to have a lifetime love of exercise there are going to be a lot more performance days ahead of you. For this reason you might as well start learning about performance at this stage.

On your performance day put some of your focus on learning. Sure, most of your focus will go into the actions that will deliver the goal but you also want to keep a conscious eye on what you can learn about performance. This learning will be an important part of determining where you will grow in the next stage of your journey.

So commit to having the perspective that your performance day is also a learning day for you. Getting to your finish line will be an amazing experience but it will also help open the doors for you to see how you can grow moving forward.

STRATEGY #9: Don't let doubt lead to bad decisions

A few years ago I was training a lady called Sam to run a marathon. Sam was a coach's dream; she was hard working, did the training that you planned for her and was a sponge for learning. As a coach you start to understand which athletes have a higher chance of achieving on the big stage, they just do everything right in preparation. Sam was one of these athletes.

Sam had set the goal of running a sub 3:10 marathon, which meant she was a strong local age group athlete. As a coach, your job is to physically and mentally prepare your athlete so they are capable of delivering on their goal. By learning about your athlete's strengths and weaknesses you gain an understanding of their ability and chances of achieving the goal they set out to achieve.

With Sam I was almost 100% certain she would achieve her goal as there was a lot of evidence to prove it. She had a history of performing on her race days, the training she had been doing for the last four months showed that she was hitting the times and intensities that she needed to run a sub 3:10 marathon, and she also had a tough mental edge. I was feeling confident for her.

There's a nervous moment for a coach who's standing at the finish line of a marathon. It's that time where the clock is ticking down to the time you know your athlete wants to achieve. You are hoping to see your athlete come around the corner and sprint to the finish line under their goal time. You want this so much because you know how hard your athlete has worked and you want them to have the amazing emotional high of achieving a tough challenge. Unfortunately on Sam's race day I didn't get to see Sam have that moment.

The clock ticked over—3:10 and there was no sight of Sam; 3:20, still no Sam; 3:45, still no Sam. Finally at 4:06 Sam came up the finishing shoot to finish her race. Three-ten was an ambitious goal so there was always a chance that Sam wouldn't achieve this goal but I would have expected her to come in somewhere between 3:08 and 3:30—4:06 was a disaster of a day.

145

Marathons can have this effect. If you get it wrong you can end up going a lot slower than you had hoped for but Sam was a seasoned runner who had consistently performed with marathons. Obviously we had gotten something wrong.

For any athlete to improve they need to do a review of their performance. This helps to reinforce what went well and where they can improve moving forward. A couple of days after Sam's marathon we caught up for her race review. There are a series of questions I work through with an athlete in this session, one of them being, 'Did you do anything on race day that took you off your plan?'.

When I asked Sam this question she looked down, like a child does when they know they have done something wrong. She said she didn't change anything on race day but two days before the race she did a two-hour run with 50 minutes of half marathon effort. I knew Sam knew doing this two days before her marathon was a bad idea. The days leading up to the marathon are about tapering, allowing the body to recharge so it can be 100% ready to perform. No running coach would advise this session two days before a key race. When I asked her what happened she said she was full of doubt. She knew that she had trained well and that I had written a good programme that showed she could achieve this goal, but when she woke up on that morning she was overwhelmed with this feeling of doubt and felt she needed to go for that run to prove to herself that she could hit the goal. As soon as she started the marathon she knew she had made a mistake as her legs were heavy and were feeling a little sore from the run two days before. She was gutted that she made such a simple mistake.

Sam is not alone in this experience. So many people make this mistake when they are aiming to achieve a goal, in any area of their life. When they experience doubt they don't trust their plan so they make bad decisions that work against them being successful.

You need to understand that you are going to experience doubt at different stages with your goal, it's all part of the game. What you can't do is be like Sam, you can't let it lead to you making stupid decisions.

With this in mind, what is the best way for you to deal with doubt? Here's a three-step method I like to use:

1. **Catch the doubt and acknowledge its presence in your life:** When you are aiming for a goal that's important to you and that you have worked hard to achieve, doubt will appear, it's all part of the process. The fact that you are experiencing doubt is something to be proud of because it represents that you are challenging and growing as a person. So if you find you are experiencing doubt, remind yourself that it's because you are challenging yourself as a person. Be proud of this.

2. **Remind yourself to stick 100% to your plan:** This is important. You want to enjoy that you have doubt because you are challenging yourself, but you don't want to respond to doubt with doubt-led actions. Once you have acknowledged that you have doubt, remind yourself that your job is to 100% stick to the plan you have in place. If you feel you need to call your mentor or coach to get their reinforcement, I guarantee that they will point you back to your plan and tell you to stay on the path.

3. **Act upon your plan:** Keep taking the actions that are in your plan: It's as simple as that. Trust and act upon it and you'll be doing the wisest thing possible.

You don't want to work so hard to achieve a goal that is so important to you and then let doubt cause you to make a bad decision that leads to you failing. Know that doubt is going to be a part of this experience but also know how to respond to it. This will keep you on the path that will give you the highest chance of success.

By the way, Sam did end up running a sub 3:10 marathon eventually, so she obviously learnt the lesson of how to deal with doubt.

Mindsets to practise for Baby Step 5

- I am learning how to achieve a fitness goal so I'll enjoy the process.

- Perfection isn't the goal, learning is.

- When I have a bad day—and I will—I'll put my focus on achieving the next session.

- I will be good at capturing the good experiences along the way and I will allow myself to own my successes.

- My performance day is a learning experience. I'll prepare as best as possible but also be aware that I will learn some valuable lessons from it.

- I will look for opportunities to use the Good On Top Of Good strategy.

- When I experience doubt I will acknowledge that feeling but I will focus on sticking to my plan.

- I will be proud that I have even reached this point in my journey.

- Feedback is important so I will be open to the feedback I get.

Workbook for Baby Step 5

Baby Step 5 does not have a defined time frame as everyone's Proud Goal will have different time requirements. The workbook for this step is there to help you be as effective as possible in your development as you move towards achieving your goal. In each Weekly Meeting go through these questions to help you get the most out of the next week.

1. What did I do well last week?

2. What do I need to reinforce for next week from the above answers?

3. What have I learnt in the last week?

4. How do I make sure I apply this learning next week?

5. Looking towards the next week, what are the key moments that I have to prepare for and how can I increase the chance of success?

6. Do I have any confusion about what I need to do at this stage?

7. Do I have any questions for my leaders/mentors?

8. What external things do I need to be aware of? (This could be identifying that work next week will be busy)

9. What's my motivational statement for this week?

10. How do I want to feel in my next Weekly Meeting?

Where to from here?

Baby Step 5 is a massive step in your journey to creating a lifetime love of exercise and doesn't have a set time frame around it as it is goal dependent. For now, most of your focus will be on applying your plan and achieving your first goal. My advice would be to come back to the book and read the next Baby Step around two weeks before the date of your goal achievement. You will need to do some planning for the next Baby Step so this will give you plenty of time.

Success in this step equals:

*   You would have consistently done the work towards achieving your first Proud Goal.

*   You would have completed your first Proud Goal!

*   You would have applied the learnings from this step and those from your leaders or mentors along the way.

*   You would have grown as a person.

- You would have experienced many physical and mental rewards.

- You'll be excited to move towards the next Baby Step.

Imagine...

What will it be like when you have achieved your goal? Imagine the benefits you will have gained and the lessons you will have learnt about yourself along the way. Also think about your journey and how this has evolved you in so many amazing ways.

You have all of this in front of you. Now go ahead and achieve your goal.

Share your Goal Achievement

Once you have achieved your first Proud Goal go to our social pages and share this with us, we'd love to see a photo too!
Use hashtag #achievedmyproudgoal

To join our social pages go to:
www.passionaboutexercise.com/social

Remember you can sign up for the Passion for Exercise course by going to:
www.passionaboutexercise.com/course

Chapter 8

How to get the most out of your achievements

It was an important race; the A race of my season. As an endurance athlete you have A, B and C races. The grading represents the importance of the race. A C race may be a small local event with a distance that is achievable with your current base fitness. A B race is where you are trying to test yourself against some of your tougher competitors and you are looking for a strong performance. But the A race is the one you commit your life to.

The A race often comes after months of hard work. It's a race where you are aiming to achieve your highest level and the chances of success are far from guaranteed; it's the race you are wanting to succeed in the most.

My A race was an Ironman where I was hoping to win my age group. The previous year I had placed fourth which qualified me for the challenging Hawaii Ironman which was an amazing race where I felt I had raced to the best of my ability. After doing the Hawaii Ironman I wanted to go back to the race where I had qualified—Ironman New Zealand—and win my age group.

The months leading up to this race were some of the most focused I had ever experienced. I was on fire, averaging over 35 hours of hard exercise every week. I had a crew of elite athletes whom I was training with and each day we would go out and try to destroy ourselves. It was such a hard time but it was also amazingly stimulating.

One problem a lot of endurance athletes have is that they can be a legendary trainer but then they don't deliver on race day. Their race performance doesn't match what their training tells them they should achieve. I knew I was fit and I knew that if I could pull off the performance my training showed was possible I had a high chance of achieving my goal. I didn't want to be the athlete who couldn't deliver on the day.

Most endurance athletes have mixed experiences on race day. There are days where you are thinking about quitting from the moment the gun goes off, to days where you have contrasting moments, moments where you feel on top of the world followed by moments where you doubt you can finish. The one we all hope for is the perfect day.

The perfect day is something special. If you are lucky as an endurance athlete you may experience a handful of these in your career. The perfect day is magic; you race feeling like you have the wind at your back all day long, when you need to push harder you seem to have energy to be able to put your foot down, and the closer you get to the finish the stronger you can push. The perfect day makes the hours and hours of hard work that goes into this crazy sport all worth it.

As I was wading into the water before the start of Ironman New Zealand I remember thinking, 'You've done the work, now put it together'. Put it together I did. I had the perfect day. From the moment the gun went off I knew it was going to be one of those special races. I had the ability to keep pushing for over nine hours.

I remember turning into the finishing shoot knowing that I had won my age group. Normally at the end of an Ironman you 'just get' to the finish line—meaning you just jog to the end—but the emotions of the perfect day, seeing my friends and family, and seeing my finish time knowing I had won my age group overtook me. Suddenly I turned into an Olympic sprinter and ran as fast as

I could to the finish line. I was overwhelmed with emotion.

After crossing the finish line and getting my finisher's medal I started walking to the post-race tent to get a massage and some food. As I was walking towards the tent I bumped into one of the top triathlon coaches in New Zealand. He had seen me come across the line and could see that I had won my age group. Looking back I still find it bizarre that he said what he said. He walked up to me and said, 'So, what's next?'. There was no 'Great work, mate', 'What a good performance', 'Well done on winning your age group'. All I got was, 'So, what's next?'.

I'll be honest, at this point the massive effort of this race was starting to hit me and my fatigue levels were pretty high and everything was becoming a bit of a blur, so I just responded with, 'I'll have to have a think about it.'

Over the next few days I couldn't stop thinking about this question. I wasn't thinking about it because it was a good question to be asked as a way of helping me grow as an athlete. I was thinking about it because I was fascinated that, in one of the most rewarding moments in my triathlon career when I was feeling on top of the world, I felt the timing of the question was atrocious. The moment straight after I had crossed the finish line and achieved a goal I had worked so hard for should only be about one thing—celebration.

I understand where the coach was coming from, he was trying to challenge me to think about a higher level, and I do believe that this type of challenge is important but when we have moments of progress and achievement we also need celebration. Celebration is like the icing on the cake, an amazing moment that unfortunately a lot of people forget to do and so miss out on this important part of the journey.

By this stage of your journey you have just achieved your first fitness goal. This is something to be embraced and celebrated, especially if we think back to where you started from. I can almost 100% guarantee that if you achieved your goal you are feeling good about yourself, proud of what you have achieved, and are probably experiencing feelings that you haven't felt in a long time. Why would we want to rush past this? By allowing yourself some time to celebrate you cement the good feeling exercise brings to your life, which makes it more appealing to keep it there for the long term.

Alongside celebration, the post-goal period has some very important components that need to be put in place. This is what Baby Step 6 is all about.

Baby Step 6: Celebrate, reflect and learn

After you achieve your goal, first you get to celebrate and then you need to put time into reflecting and learning from the experience. If you get this part right you will be excited about your next step and have a good understanding of where you can grow as you progress forward. That's what you are going to do now.

Challenge for Baby Step 6

To book in time to celebrate and then to book in time to reflect and learn.

Rules for Baby Step 6

RULE #1: Plan some form of celebration

The first thing I want to acknowledge is that we are all different. Some people want to have an entire birthday week while others are happy to have a low-key drink with their partner or a friend. What celebration means to one person can be different to another so I encourage you to do the form of celebration that is aligned to you. The most important thing is that you plan it.

Make a commitment to giving yourself the time and space to celebrate. This is like putting icing on an already delicious cake. You've achieved your goal, now you can embrace all of the goodness that comes with this achievement.

RULE #2: Plan time for reflection and learning

You know how sometimes in life we have things we know we should do but we procrastinate? This is understandable when it's an area that we don't see a lot of value in, like that project at work that is not stimulating, but often we can put the things off that have a massive return on their time investment. One of these areas is your post-challenge reflection and learning.

When you fail to do your post-challenge reflection and learning you miss an amazing opportunity to see what you did well and want to reinforce moving forward, but you are also missing the chance to see where you can grow and where you need to challenge yourself in the next stage of your evolution. So many people never progress because they don't spend the time discovering where they need to grow next. We don't want you to be this person.

You want to be like a high-level athlete, you want to reflect, review and learn from this experience so you can reinforce your good stuff and see where you want to put your energy as you move forward. Don't see this as a chore, see it as an exciting opportunity to learn a higher level of yourself.

Strategies to use in Baby Step 6

STRATEGY #1: Find the best way for you to celebrate, and plan it

When you get to the end point of your challenge there's a high chance that you will feel a massive sense of achievement. This is an amazing feeling and you want to embrace this as much as possible. In many ways this moment is enough of a reward for your effort but as a part of this journey we do want you to have a special celebration that sits on top of this.

This is where you want to know yourself. Celebrating can be done in many different ways. It might be that you have dinner with the people that were a part of your journey, it could be that you buy yourself new training fashion, it could be as simple as a post on social media. The key to your celebration is that it feels right for you and that you actually do it.

You may want to plan your celebration before your challenge event. You can use this as a motivator along the way. It can be, 'If I achieve my goal I'm going to go for a treat weekend away'. Using your celebration as a motivator is a good tool.

When the time comes to actually celebrate, make sure you embrace it. This is about you not dismissing your moment in the sun. Allow yourself to feel on top of the world, you deserve it.

STRATEGY #2: Make the people who have supported you feel valued

I did the sport of Ironman for about six years of my life and in this time I put a lot of time and energy into trying to be the best athlete I could be, but I would never have achieved what I did if I didn't have an amazing group of people around me.

When I completed my last Ironman I wrote a race report about my race. In this report I acknowledged that this was my last Ironman race. I wanted to spend time acknowledging and thanking all the people who were a part of my time in the sport. I wanted to give back to these people with words that showed them how much I valued them. Here's what I wrote:

> Since this is kind of my goodbye to Ironman there are a few people I want to thank. Fred Harding, Graham Ewing, Neil Graham, Albert Boyce and Adrianne Shaw—these guys all gave in very special ways.
>
> My sponsors over the years: Genius Bikes, Scotty Browns, Blue Seventy, Fifth Element, Coffees of Hawaii and Bolle sunglasses.
>
> Everybody who financially gave through supporting my fundraising to help me achieve my goals. Your gifts—small or large—meant so much more than the dollar you gave. Plus the people who helped coordinate a lot of the fundraising—you gave your time and energy to help me achieve my goals! That still blows my mind.
>
> My girlfriends over this time, Rae and Annelies. Ironman

triathletes aren't the easiest partners to be with but both of you were great at supporting an obsessed young man—you both were amazing!

The Ironman Talk community. What started as a silly training idea has turned into such a valuable part of my life. I never get sick of the emails of support for my goals and the show.

Members from the Christchurch gym, without knowing it you helped pull me through many tough days. Some of the loveliest people there are.

My homestays, people who open up their home and let you make it yours! I will pay this forward and try to maintain the high standards you all set.

The people who I have trained with over the years. There's something about being around people who thrive on a challenge and know how to breathe the air of life.

'Coach' John Newsom. His passion for triathlon and willingness to share his knowledge is amazing. We've shared some great experiences together. You are a real mate.

My friends. This sport has helped me realise how important you are. Thanks for being there for me. A special mention must go to Dunk, Fraser, Geoff and Kate. These guys would come from all around New Zealand at a high cost just to yell at me on the side lines, plus do a little Ironman drinking ;-)

Mum, Dad and Shelley. I have to admit I'm getting a little emotional right now! I can honestly say that I have the best family in the world! Their love for me is unbelievable. I could achieve nothing without them. Everything I have ever achieved is because I know these guys are there in my heart. I will never forget riding in the middle of nowhere in a race seeing a crazy bunch of people (often dressed up in the craziest gear) making the most noise of any supporters out there and thinking with pride 'that's my family!'

Tyla Jade Eyles (my daughter). If anyone has had to

put up with someone being tired, it's you. I love you more than you'll ever know. I'll never forget how you would go and get a blanket when you would see that I had crashed on the couch or how you knew 'watching a movie' together would mean I would fall asleep within five minutes but you would cuddle up and enjoy being with your dad. You are very special!

Lastly, everybody who ever sent me an email, showed interest in or followed my progress. I truly believe that people are good and you always showed that side of yourself to me.

In our sport there's a phrase that goes 'one-and-done', for the people who only compete in one Iron distance race. A wise triathlete once said, 'It's a pity that those people don't gain the true life lessons that competing in Ironman for a few years brings'. I leave this passion of mine having learnt those lessons, what a journey!

I hope that the people who helped me on my journey felt amazing about themselves as they read this. I wanted them to feel this way. These people gave to me in so many ways, the least I could do is repay them by showing them how much this meant to me.

Your celebration is partly about you feeling great about your achievement but it's also about making those who have supported you feel like they are a big part of it as well. You want to express how much their support means to you. You want them to feel awesome for being the people that they are.

Commit time in your celebration period to give the love back. You can do this in the way that feels right to you. From my experience one of the best feelings in life is to make someone else feel good about themselves so I'm sure you will love including this as part of your celebrations.

STRATEGY #3: Get a keepsake that represents this achievement

This strategy is optional but I do find it can be effective. One of the coolest parts of finishing a well-organised running race is that you get a medal once you cross the finish line. This is another one of those 'icing on the cake' moments. You are already feeling great because you finished and now you get a medal that represents this. This keepsake is something that represents an achievement that you are proud of and it's a reminder of a moment in your life that you are proud of.

Not all challenges are going to have medals but that doesn't mean you can't have a keepsake. I have a friend who likes doing crazy cycling challenges, like riding around Australia in its entirety! The challenges weren't organised events so there was no practical reward that came with completing it, but what he did do was buy a piece of art from a local artist where he did his challenge. He has a room in his house that is filled with all the different pieces of art he has collected and each one represents a different challenge in his life. I imagine every time he goes into that room so many amazing memories are triggered.

If your challenge provides a keepsake, put it somewhere that you see often. If it doesn't, be creative and come up with something that will represent this important moment in your life and act as a reminder of this special time.

STRATEGY #4: Plan time to do your reflection and learning and do it soon after your challenge

I was coaching a guy called Jim who was wanting to achieve a sub 3:30 marathon, a goal that he had been striving to achieve for years but had never quite gotten there. He'd done over 20 marathons and before we started working together his best time was 3:41. He loved marathons but was always disappointed because he never performed to the level that he thought he could. He believed he could run under 3:30 but each time he'd blow up in the last 5-10km of the race and miss out on his goal.

When Jim contacted me he was at his wits end. He was desperate to achieve his dream goal and after doing some run testing it became clear that Jim should be able to achieve his goal; his results showed a sub 3:30 was well within his ability. Something was wrong and it was my job to help him fix it.

Jim was a coach's dream, he was motivated, responsive, open to learning, and was hard working. Over the next five months we worked on a plan to help him achieve his goal. This plan addressed not just the physical training but also included his rest and recharge strategies, it developed his mental game, created his perfect nutrition strategy and got him practising his race tactics.

I loved working with Jim because whenever I asked something of him, he would do it. I remember I gave him a mental skills course which required homework to be done each Monday. Every Monday morning the first email I would get would be from Jim with his homework. His level of commitment showed how much this goal meant to him.

All of his work paid off because on his race day he finished the race in 3:26:26. Watching him coming into the finishing shoot was the coolest thing to see. Jim was overcome with emotion and started crying as he crossed the finish line—he'd done it. He'd achieved a goal that he'd work for years to achieve.

Two days after the race, when the celebrations had died down, I sent Jim an email that included my post-race report document. This is a document I send to athletes with the sole purpose of learning and reflecting. I let Jim know I would like it back by the following Monday so we could do some work on his future goals. Jim being Jim, I expected to get this document back on the same day or the following day, but that didn't happen. The following Monday came along and there was no email in my inbox. I flicked Jim a text on Monday to see if he had sent it through. He called me back to say sorry but he hadn't gotten around to it. Here was my 'easy to coach' athlete who did everything to be successful now shifting away from the level that had created success for him.

Spending time reflecting and learning from our challenge experience is so important but I've learnt it's something that people have every intention of doing but often don't get around to it. Once we have achieved the goal we allow ourselves to release the 'importance valve' off a little bit. We let things slip because we have achieved what we set out to do and although understandable, by neglecting to do your post-challenge reflection and learning you are missing out on one of the most important tools needed for your evolution.

If you want to continue to grow in this area the best time to learn is close to when you did the challenge. More importantly, if you give yourself time and have a practical process to go through you'll have a document to use as you move towards your next goal. This document will guide the choices you make on where and how you will develop yourself.

The most important thing is that you commit time for this process and do it soon after you have completed your challenge. It's ok to take a couple days off to celebrate and unwind but you want to have this work done within seven days of your challenge completion. Make this commitment and you'll be fast-forwarding your future process.

STRATEGY #5: Get your leader/mentor involved

Highly experienced people have the ability to see things others can't and have a higher level of understanding and knowledge. Your personal self reflection is important but when you add your mentor's insight to this process you are getting a wise soul guiding you. They have the ability to open you up to different growth points in areas that you may not have thought of or seen.

Aim to include your leader or mentor in this process even if there's a cost—it's a great investment in your future growth.

STRATEGY #6: Have a series of reflective/learning questions to work through

If you are lucky, your leader or mentor may have a post-challenge document for you to work through and if they do, it will be a series of questions that will help you see what you have done well, what to reinforce moving forward and where there are areas for improvement.

Here's an example of what I send to my clients after a race:

Event: ————————————————————————

Date: —————————————————————————

Distance: ———————————————————————

Result: ————————————————————————

- How well did you train for this race?

- What was the best thing you did in your training?

- What do you feel are the two most important areas for you to improve in your training?

- On a scale of 1 to 10 (1 = poor, 10 = exceptional), how would you rate this performance? Why did you rank it as such?

- What was your travel itinerary to the event? Did this affect your performance (positively or negatively)?

- How were the stress levels in your life in the days before the race?

- How were your sleeping patterns in the days before the race?

- How were your eating habits in the days before the race?

- What were the weather conditions for the race? What specific preparations did you make for these conditions (hydration, clothing, etc.)? Were these preparations adequate?

- What was your warm-up routine for the race? Was it effective? If not, what would have been more effective?

- What were you thinking about on the start line? Did this help or hurt your performance?

- On a scale of 1 to 10 (1 = poor, 10 = exceptional), what was your motivation level for this race? Why did you rank it as such?

- What was your nutrition plan for the race? How well did you execute the plan? Could the plan be improved? How?

- What was your hydration plan for the race? How well did you execute the plan? Could the plan be improved? If so, how?

- What was your pacing strategy for the race? How well did you execute the strategy? (List your mile/lap splits, if applicable). What do your splits show about your execution?

- What decisions did you make before or during the race that helped your performance?

- What decisions did you make before or during the race that did not help your performance?

- What motivation strategies did you use in the race? Were they effective?

- Anything else about the race (positive or negative) that you feel is important?

- What are the key areas for you to improve in your next race?

While these questions are specifically focused on an endurance running race you can see how they can get someone thinking to a deeper level about their entire experience. The answers that come from working through these questions will give a deeper insight into performance and help develop where growth can be made moving forward.

Come up with a series of questions that will work for the challenge that you did. They may cover topics like your training routine, your performance (both physical and mental), or external factors. This leads into the next strategy.

STRATEGY #7: Be honest and realistic about your performance and look for the detail

There's no value in reflecting on your performance if you aren't honest with yourself and this can go one of two ways. You can put rose-tinted glasses on and paint the experience as perfect or beat yourself up for everything you got wrong. What you are looking for in your reflection/learning time is a realistic representation of how you performed. There are going to be good areas and areas to improve on. You want to be honest and look at the facts.

A good tool to use here is to look at the performance assessment as if you were assessing someone else. It's like having a third eye look at your performance, one where you don't have a personal emotional attachment to it. This technique will allow you to keep to the facts.

The more you can create an honest, realistic and deeper representation of your performance the better you'll be able to set your future goals. With this work in place you'll be on the right track as you move further down your exercise path.

STRATEGY #8: Expand your reflection and learning to the whole training period

Performance day is the peak moment in any journey but it's the day-to-day work that's just as important to your success. If you don't practise your basketball shots in training there's less chance you'll make the shot in the big game, or if you don't do your long run in training for a half marathon there's a high chance that you will fade in the last part of the run. During your learning and reflection time you are not just looking at your performance day, you are looking at the whole period of training leading up to that day too.

It's interesting watching my wife after she has completed a running goal and then starts to set her next one. She always finds something in her training that she's looking to improve. It might be an area of technique to work on or tweaks to her training nutrition. Her next areas of focus come from reflecting on the training she has just completed.

It's so important to reflect and learn from your entire training period—not just the finale!

STRATEGY #9: At the end of this reflection period identify areas for improvement

I've always been a small business owner and one of the challenges this brings is that you are limited on time, money and resources. There are so many things that I would love to do with my business and there are so many opportunities in front of me but there are also many problems that my team and I have to solve. One of the biggest questions a small business owner needs to ask themselves is, 'What is the right problem/project for me and my team to be working on right now?'

This is a powerful question because many small business owners put a lot of their limited time, money and resources into solving problems that don't need to be solved then and there. Often they can wait, they need to be acknowledged as something that needs attention, but a solution isn't required imminently.

Problems arise because the focus is moved away from issues and opportunities that are real right now and are neglected. Many businesses have gone under because their focus was on the wrong thing and the question, 'What is the right problem/project to be solving right now?' wasn't asked.

At this stage of your fitness journey you are a newbie. It's exciting that you have achieved your first goal and there are so many possibilities around where you can grow. What's important is that you have a clear understanding of what the wisest next step is for your growth so this question relates well to where you are right now: 'What is the next wise step in your journey for you right now?'.

Consider things like your current skill levels, character traits, and ability to be successful within the time frame you have. By thinking about these things and using my question you'll have clear answers on what you need to work on next.

Ideally your next challenge should have one or two key growth areas and these will be the right level of 'stretch' for your current ability. By being a master of your reflection/learning time and using that small business owner question you will have a clear idea of what these areas will be.

New Zealand's greatest male Ironman triathlete of all time is a man called Cameron Brown. He's one of only a handful of professional athletes to win the same Ironman race ten times; it's a phenomenal achievement in such a hard sport. I remember interviewing Cameron years ago where he beat his record at Ironman New Zealand. In the interview Cameron told me that before the race he went back and read all of his post-race reports from all of his years of racing and doing this gave him confidence. He also told me that this process had reminded him of where he needed to focus in this performance.

My interview with Cam showed the level that a high performer plays at. He had all of his race reports from all of his years of racing. When you get to Cam's level you are looking for the centimetre gains in performance. His reports were a massive tool in finding those centimetres.

By implementing this tool and making it a habit within your goal periods you are setting up the fastest, wisest path forward and who knows, if you keep on this path maybe you'll be like Cam Brown in the future, looking for the centimetres in your performance.

Mindsets to practise for Baby Step 6

- Committing time and energy to celebration, learning and reflection is the most valuable use of my time.

- It's good for me to enjoy celebrating my growth. I'm allowed to enjoy it so I will embrace it.

- My celebration should include those who supported me along the way. I will make them feel special and valued.

- The best way to find my path forward is to learn from my

experience and be honest about where I can grow.

- By doing the work in this Baby Step I'm going to have more moments of growth and celebration in my life.

Workbook for Baby Step 6

Your celebration, reflection and learning period should all be done within ten days, at the most two weeks, of your goal day. You can do some of it before your goal day. Plan it in your Weekly Meeting, this way your celebration, reflection and learning time will be in your diary!

Here are the questions to explore at this time:

1. What is the best way for me to celebrate that feels right for me?

2. Do I need to set up anything for this celebration?

3. How do I make sure I do this?

4. How will I include the people that have been a part of this journey as a part of my celebration?

5. When is the best time for me to get my reflection/learning done? (Book this time into your diary).

6. What are the questions I need to work through that will help me gain the most insight from my experience? (You may want to ask your mentor about this).

7. What attitude will serve me best when I do my reflection and learning?

8. How do I make sure I have a clear understanding of where I can grow next at the end of my reflecting/learning session?

Where to from here?

This Baby Step has a short time frame and while there is work to be done within it, the best approach would be to read the next Baby Step after you have completed your goal and are in your celebration and reflection time.

The next moment in this journey is so important in setting the long-term fitness habit in place so remember it needs to be done within a short time period after your goal day. If you get this done in the Weekly Meeting following your goal completion day you can then devote your next Weekly Meeting to starting the work on Baby Step 7.

I know, there's a lot of self work over this period but make sure you stick at it because if you get this next moment right you'll be flying with your fitness for the long term.

Success in this step equals:

- You will have celebrated your journey in a way that was aligned to you and the people who were a part of your journey.

- You will have a deep understanding of what you did well and where you can improve moving forward.

- You will have two to three areas for improvement set in place for the next challenge.

- You will feel proud of yourself because you have done the small things that a lot of people don't do.

Imagine...

If you had not only completed your first fitness goal but were celebrating your achievement with the people who were part of your experience, imagine how you would feel. Then imagine if you had learnt the key lessons that will help you continue to evolve your exercise journey and you were excited to take on the next challenge. That's what this Baby Step is about. This can be a reality for you soon.

Share your Celebration

When you're celebrating your achievement, take a photo and share it on our social media page!
Use hashtag #mycelebration

To join our social pages go to:
www.passionaboutexercise.com/social

Remember you can sign up for the Passion for Exercise course by going to:
www.passionaboutexercise.com/course

Chapter 9

How to avoid going backwards after making progress

I've always been good at giving compliments. I strongly believe that if you see someone has improved or has done something good you should let them know that you are impressed by them. When I give compliments I aim to be specific so instead of just saying, 'You did well in today's run', I like to say, 'I love how in the last set you showed grit and hard working character traits to push through'. This next level of detail gives the person receiving it acknowledgement that you are genuine and really have noticed that they have done something great.

Being a compliment giver has its rewards because people like feeling good about themselves, so when you give a compliment you tend to get a nice version of that person coming back to you. This is a good thing to have in your life but there are times when giving a compliment can lead to an awkward interaction.

A few years ago I was at the shopping mall on a rainy afternoon. As I was walking around the mall I saw someone in the distance whose face looked familiar but I couldn't figure out what the connection was. I knew this person but for the life of me I couldn't figure out how I knew them. When I sat down for lunch I saw this person again but this time they weren't off in the distance, they were walking towards me with a big smile on their face, they were coming to have a chat.

Luckily for me when he was about ten metres away it clicked. I had worked with this person years earlier and it's fair to say that I had a good relationship with him, we were good workmates and he was not the type of person I would normally forget! You might be thinking that I'm not a very good friend but in fairness to me he had gone through a massive change. My old workmate had lost weight and I don't mean a little bit of weight, he had probably lost over 40kg.

I asked if he had time to have lunch and over the next hour we caught up on life, told old work stories and spent a lot of time talking about his weight loss journey. I was so impressed with what my workmate had gone through. Being a fitness professional I have a good understanding of how hard a weight loss journey can be.

As we were wrapping up our conversation I gave my friend a compliment, one of those detailed ones I like to give. I told him how proud I was and that the character and discipline required to achieve this is massive, that he is an inspiration to me and many others. I could see that my friend valued my words.

Life went on and our interaction seemed to be a one-off experience, until around two years later. I was standing in a queue at the bank and when I turned around, guess who was behind me? My old workmate. This time I recognised him straight away, not because I remembered him from the mall but because he was the physical version I had worked with all of those years ago. Unfortunately my friend had put all of the weight back on.

You know how sometimes during a conversation there's an obvious elephant in the room? This was one of those moments. I've never judged an overweight person; while they may have weight struggles I would be a fool to limit my experience of them because of it. But when I turned around and saw my friend I was slightly shocked and my facial expression revealed that I had noticed his weight gain. He made a joke about putting the weight back on. I felt terrible that my look had made him feel bad so I quickly tried to change the subject and asked how he'd been. He took my lead and avoided the weight gain discussion. As we parted ways I felt terrible that I had made my friend feel bad about himself and I decided I would get in touch to see if he would like to have a chat about what had happened.

I approached the catch up as a fitness professional who has helped many people to grow with health and fitness. Our discussion was so valuable to me because it taught me some of the most important lessons about creating and sustaining change in your life.

In my view, the weight loss journey is one of the most challenging journeys people can face as it requires behavioural change. With weight loss you can't go cold turkey and just quit eating, like an alcoholic can with drinking. You have to face choices around food several times a day—everyday. If you have been on a weight loss journey that has taken six months to achieve your goal you have had to face thousands and thousands of decisions requiring a huge amount of effort to get you to this place. That's why it's so impressive when people can achieve this.

When we look at the typical weight loss journey it goes a bit like this: You get to the point where you are sick of being overweight and decide you need to change. This moment can be triggered by many things, like health concerns, being dissatisfied within yourself, or feeling that your life is limited due to your weight. This motivation for change needs a plan so the next step is to find a plan that will help you achieve your weight-loss goal.

Ultimately a plan is a set of behaviours that, if maintained for a certain period of time, will achieve the outcome you desire. Let's say you are 20kg overweight so you search for a weight loss solution. A good plan will cover the nutrition choices you need to make but it will also address the emotional, psychological and physical aspects of your journey. After some research you find your plan.

The plan you commit to will:

- reduce calories across your day
- change the types of foods you are eating
- get you moving more
- help you develop mental strategies that create success in all aspects of weight loss

Your plan has the goal of you losing 20kg over a ten-month period. Because you are highly motivated and disciplined and have stayed focused throughout the ten-month period, you experience success. Ten months later you are looking in the mirror feeling super proud of yourself. Sure, you look better but you also have more energy, have more confidence in yourself and are putting yourself out there for more experiences in your life. You are proud of yourself because you know how much character it took to get to this place.

What I find interesting is the next moment—the moment after you achieve the goal of losing 20kg. This is where we can return to my friend from the mall. I wanted to see if I could help him with my fitness professional hat on. We arranged to go for a walk together at one of my favourite local trails.

We both knew the reason for the catch up so once we started walking we got straight onto the topic. My friend told me that when we bumped into each other at the mall he had just achieved his weight loss goal and was at the peak of his journey. He said if I had asked him if there was any chance that he would put the weight back on he would have said there was no chance, he had found his formula for weight loss and he was going to stick to it.

I asked him where he went wrong and he said it wasn't one big thing, it was more like there was a slow slippage back to his old behaviours.

When he was losing weight he had a rule that he would only drink alcohol on a Saturday night. Before his weight loss journey he would drink three to four times a week but wasn't an excessive drinker and reducing his drinking seemed like an easy win. But once he'd achieved his goal he let that rule slip. A couple of Fridays later he had a work function and thought it would be okay to have a drink. Then the following weekend he let himself have a couple of drinks while watching some sport. He'd walked right back through the door to his old behaviours and within a month was back to drinking three to four times a week.

And it wasn't just with alcohol, his food choices also slipped back. His portion sizes started increasing and he slowly slipped away from exercise to the point where he wasn't exercising at all.

My friend's experience is one that many people go through. If we go back to the definition of a plan for change, a plan is a set of behaviours that if maintained for a certain period of time will achieve the outcome you desire. My friend's plan worked but the important moment for sustainable long-term change didn't happen and this is because once he had achieved his goal he slowly slipped back to his old behaviours.

This is such an important lesson for you right now on your journey. The goal of this book isn't to help you have a 'one-off' fitness experience where you achieve a goal that you are proud of. It's to help you have a lifetime love of exercise where it's a sustainable part of your everyday life. But right now you are in a moment where you can start to cement exercise in your life or you can slowly slip away from it and go back to that old version of yourself.

The thing is, just about everyone who achieves behavioural change successfully tells themselves they will maintain these behaviours. My friend had every intention of limiting his alcohol to just Saturday nights but once the goal or focus was removed the slippage began.

With this in mind we need to acknowledge that having good intentions of maintaining good behaviours after the goal is achieved is a bad strategy. Instead, we need to put good strategies in place to keep you evolving. That's where the next Baby Step comes into play.

Baby Step 7: Set a new goal that is the perfect next step in your fitness evolution

If you are undertaking the journey of this book, you have just achieved your fitness goal. This may be the first fitness goal you have achieved in years, which is amazing, but if you don't get this Baby Step right you could wake up in a few months from now back to where you were before you started this journey. I don't want this for you and I can 100% guarantee that you don't want this either. We are aiming to create a lifetime love of exercise so it's important that you get this Baby Step right.

Challenge for Baby Step 7

To set a new goal using all of the successful goal-setting strategies you have used so far which will be the wisest next step in your fitness journey.

Rules for Baby Step 7

RULE #1: Set this goal two weeks after achieving your first fitness challenge

The post-challenge celebration, learning and reflection time is really important. It's also important that after you come off a focused training period you allow yourself a bit of down time. A lot of people struggle with this as they can feel a little bit lost and have a lack of direction. This makes sense, going from working hard with focus to then achieving the goal and no longer having a plan or focus ahead can be tough. In endurance sport we call this the post-race blues.

The first thing to acknowledge is that it's ok to feel this way, it's normal. Use this post-challenge time to relax, recharge, do your celebration and learning work, and to recover. This time is important as it can increase the desire to set a new goal; so when it comes time to look at 'what next' you have the energy to do it.

Setting your new goal is an important step in this journey and you need to do it within a short period of time after achieving your first challenge, no more than two weeks after completion of your last goal. This time frame allows you to have a week of down time but also keeps you on track with your fitness.

Why two weeks? Slipping back into our old habits can happen quickly so a two-week time frame is a good amount of time to recover without letting things slip too much. I've also learnt that after two weeks of downtime people have an itch to start something new; we want to capitalise on this.

RULE #2: Make the goal the perfect next 'stretch' in your evolution

Years ago, a guy called Cieran came and stayed with me for four months while he was preparing to race an Ironman in New Zealand. At that time my flatmates and I were in our mid-twenties and he was in his fifties so he was a funny fit for the household. He was a man who was disciplined, well-read, and enjoyed the simple things in life while the rest of us in the house were your typical 'twenty-somethings'. The nice thing about the contrast in age and priorities in our lives was that we both influenced each other in good ways.

I've always played music and at that time one of my best mates would come around every week and we would have a guitar jam session. They were fun nights where we would play and sing songs together. Cieran wasn't a musician but it was clear that he enjoyed our jam sessions so I asked him if he would like me to teach him how to play the guitar, to which he replied 'yes'.

I had a spare guitar so I gave it to him and taught him his first song. I decided to teach him a really basic song that I knew he would love. Looking back it was a great first Proud Goal for his guitar playing because it was achievable and he would be proud to play it when he got good at it.

Cieran wasn't working while he was in New Zealand doing his training so he had a bit of spare time each day which was now filled with him practising his song like crazy. After a week of practising he was able to play it at a very good beginner level.

177

Don't get me wrong, he was far from perfect but he was able to play it to a level where people would know what song it was.

Because of his discipline and early success I decided it was time for Cieran to have his second lesson. This is where my lack of understanding around helping people grow was exposed, which ended up in Cieran quitting.

Because Cieran had been so good at practising and had got on top of his first song so quickly, I thought I'd give him a much harder song in his next lesson. Looking back, the next song I gave him was three to four steps above his current ability. This was a total failure. Cieran had great character traits, he was hard-working and disciplined, but his skill level was way too low for the challenge that I had put in front of him. I had set Cieran up to fail, and fail he did.

Three days after our second lesson I noticed that Cieran wasn't practising the guitar any more. I checked in to see why he had stopped and he told me the new song was too hard. Instantly I realised my mistake so I offered to teach him a new, easier song, but Cieran had lost heart and told me that it was okay, he was happy reading his books.

This experience taught me so much about how to help people develop. When we are looking to grow, the 'stretch' needs to be stimulating and realistic. In my keenness I tried to stretch Cieran too much which led to him breaking. We don't want this to happen to you at this stage of your journey.

Your next goal needs to be the perfect 'stretch' in your fitness evolution. The perfect stretch considers things like:

- Your current fitness
- Your current skill level
- Your motivational skills
- Your mental game

When you consider these areas and look at the time frame for your next goal it's good to think about what is the right stretch for you. What's the right next step in your development and fitness evolution.

When I think about my 5km running group, once our runners have achieved their first Proud Goal of running 5km you may think that the next obvious step is to aim for 10km. While we do have a stepping stone system for our runners for this next step to 10km we actually have an in-between step which sits between their first 5km run and then aiming to run 10km. We call this our 'Return to 5km' programme. This programme understands that these people can run 5km but that they need to develop more continuous running, the ability to handle some entry level intensity in their running and also develop more self confidence within themselves before they aim to run 10km.

Our Return to 5km programme loses the walk/run training, it has sets of intensity in the programme and it gets them running 8km by the end of the programme. At the end of the eight weeks of training they come back and run 5km again with the goal of beating the time they did the first time, which they all smash. From here they are ready to start their 10km running goal.

Our Return to 5km programme is a perfect stretch goal for our runners. It understands where they need to be developed and gives them the right pathway to do this.

This is what you need for your next goal. You are looking for the perfect stretch, a stretch that will allow you to be successful while developing the tools and skills you need as you evolve on your fitness journey. This Baby Step may be the most important in the whole journey of this book because if you can achieve your second fitness goal you are cementing that exercise is a part of your identity and life. For this reason choosing the right stretch goal is of utmost importance.

RULE #3: The goal needs to take you deeper into 'non-exercise' parts of your fitness journey

If we use the metaphor of a tree, at this stage you are a seedling that has sprouted and has begun to put some roots into the ground on your fitness journey. Sure, we can look at just the physical here but we also want to look at the other parts of a fitness/healthy lifestyle that you want to deepen the roots of. These include being more connected with your community and doing the things that your tribe does, and evolving your personal processes around the habits that create a healthier you.

Let's go deeper into each of these.

Being more connected with your community and doing the things that your tribe does

I fundamentally believe that the more connection we have with others and the more we feel we belong, the more successful we are with exercise. Remember Baby Step 3: Find and commit to the right exercise world for you. If you have been following the process of this book you'll have found your community and they will have been a big part of the success of your first Proud Goal. As you deepen your exercise roots you want to deepen your connections and belonging.

For this reason your next goal should aim to deepen your connection with your tribe. There will be the training sessions but it's also about committing to the social aspects of your community, like going for coffee after the session, or going and supporting other people when they are achieving their goals or helping out with other aspects of your community. Making a commitment to this side of exercise creates a stronger connection to your community and your movement.

Another thing to think about is, how do you do more of what your tribe does? A good example of this is the gear you wear. A basketball tribe has a certain look, so does a running tribe, so does an MMA tribe. This is a good thing because it represents belonging. Sure, you want to be able to express yourself in ways that are true to you but understanding what your tribe does and finding the right fit for you within this is one of the greatest ways to deepen your exercise roots. Be proud of being part of your tribe and don't be afraid to show the world this.

Evolving your personal processes around the habits that create a healthier you

By this stage you'll have learnt valuable lessons about fitness that have nothing to do with the actual physical exercise you are doing; things like planning, mental preparation and communication with your support network. Looking back on my most demanding physical challenges where I trained hard for a certain period of time, success during this time required a 'higher level of self' in all areas of my life. I had to be an amazing planner, I used my mental tools to the highest level, I had communicated with detail to my support network, I created perfect recharge strategies (like meditation and good sleep habits), and many other personal processes.

I've learnt that the higher the goal, the more I need to be on top of my personal processes in my whole life. We want to be looking to evolve our personal processes as we grow and this is what I want you to consider as you set your next goal. Sure, the goal is about a fitness/physical challenge but where can you develop yourself in your personal processes as you work towards this?

You may be a terrible planner which means you lack a bit of consistency with your training, or you have bad bedtime habits which leads to you being tired and lacking energy for your exercise. What are the areas for you? With this goal you could aim to improve one or two things about the areas you identify.

With the areas you identify, think about the perfect stretch for the time period you'll be working on this for. For example, if you want to work on your planning skills, spend 10-15 minutes every night planning out everything you need for exercise the next day. This goal isn't about you becoming the world's most detailed planner, it's about creating a realistic goal that is the right stretch in your planning development.

By the end of this goal your nightly planning habit will be in place and then you can look towards the next stage of your development.

If you continue on this fitness journey you are going to achieve goals you can't even fathom right now. When you get to that place you'll need to be a higher version of yourself in all areas of your life. Developing your personal processes now is so important but it will also help you be more successful on this stage of your journey.

Strategies to use in Baby Step 7

STRATEGY #1: After you have achieved your first Proud Goal, book in your next goal-setting session

After you have completed your first Proud Goal and are working through your celebration/reflection period, book a time in your calendar where you will set your next goal. This needs to be within two weeks of completing your first goal. Remember what I talked about earlier, you need some down time but don't wait too long, you don't want to slip back to your old self.

Be mindful of when you book this into your calendar. A goal-setting session takes effort, you need the time and space to be able to do the thinking that allows you to find the right goal. You also need to be in the right mindspace, a space where you can think deeply about your goals. When you book in your time make sure it's when you'll have the energy required.

By committing to this session you are making a commitment to staying on your new path in life. Book it in for the right time, around two weeks after achieving your goal, and you are setting yourself up for success.

STRATEGY #2: Evolve your goal-setting process

If you go back and look at my goal-setting books over the years you'll see that my process has evolved. There are some aspects that have stayed the same, some things have disappeared and there are some parts that are new.

For example, right from the start I have always had the question, 'Who will help me achieve this goal and how can they help me?', but I didn't use the question 'What do I have to give up to achieve this goal?'. I used to put detailed 'timestamps' on when I should have achieved certain steps of a goal but I found that I could never get these right. They weren't useful in my process so I dropped them.

The reason my goal-setting process has evolved is that every time I sit down the first thing I ask myself is, 'Can I evolve how I set my goals?'. This isn't looking at the actual goals I am setting, it's looking at how I set them. This question makes me see what has worked and what hasn't. It lets me think about adding new strategies to my goal-setting process and this is a good thing for you to do in your goal-setting time.

If we are going to set goals we want to do them in the most effective way possible. This means we are increasing our chance of actually achieving them. By spending this time working on the question, 'How can I evolve how I set my goals?' you will evolve your process which will lead to a higher level of success for you.

STRATEGY #3: Use all of the tools and strategies that you have used up to this point

There's no need to go into detail here as we have covered a lot of these topics already so I'll just list strategies and tools that you want to make sure you continue to use:

- Use your mentors to help guide you with your goal.

- Make it another Proud Goal that is realistic for your current ability.

- Make sure the goal will realistically fit into your life.

- Determine what you need to communicate with your world about how they can help you.

- Stay focused on only achieving your next goal.

- Be process focused.

- Look at how you can use your success formula and how you can evolve this.

- Understand what your Bad Day strategies will be.

- Keep building evidence of positive exercise experiences and in your ability.

- Use your challenge/growth mindset.

- Keep evolving how you get feedback.

- Get better at using the Good on Top of Good strategy.

- Keep learning.

STRATEGY #4: If possible, choose a goal that naturally deepens the connections with your community

Each year my running business trains our half marathon group, RaceTeam, for four different half marathon events. Each of these events has something different about them. There's the big local race, our hard winter hill race in our local area, the out-of-town off-road race and the out-of-town big event race. Because all of these groups train three times a week for ten weeks leading up to the race they have amazing camaraderie and connection, which is a powerful part of their journey. Feeling that you are working towards a goal with others gives you so much motivation.

Our team training helps deepen the connection between our runners but there's another thing we do that takes this even further; it's the races we do out of town.

When we travel to an event over a weekend our people have so many shared experiences along the way. Sure, they all get to complete an important race that they had trained so hard for but there's more than that. A lot of them will travel to the race together, share accommodation, come to our post-race function and then head out for a fun night together. They will celebrate the success with the rest of their crew before, during and after the race.

All of these moments create deeper connections; the memories, stories, the laughs, the support of each other, the celebrations.

When you have this type of experience with your people you create a deeper sense of belonging and this makes you want to stay in your fitness world. When you get to this level you hardly ever have to motivate yourself to go and train because you just want to be with your community.

If possible, when you are setting your next goal see if it can sit in line with something your community is doing. It might be a trip away to an event, a competition that everyone is aiming for, or it could even be a team event where you work with others to achieve a goal. If you can find the perfect goal that sits within something your community is doing, you will be setting yourself up to experience the next level of motivation.

Baby Step 7 is important because if you nail this step you are moving from being someone who has a 'one-off fitness experience' to being someone who has a lifetime love of exercise. As I've mentioned earlier, in my mind this is the most important step because if you get this one right you are cementing exercise as a part of your long-term future.

Side Note:

As we move into the next Baby Step we won't be working on you achieving the goal in this step. I do want you to achieve this goal and having it as this Baby Step was really important because we need you to get back on your fitness wagon in the right way. The next few Baby Steps are about your long-term fitness life. So while the focus of this book shifts you still want to put your fitness energy into achieving this goal.

Mindsets to practise for Baby Step 7

- Setting my next goal within two weeks of my goal completion will set me up for a successful fitness future.

- I want to find the perfect stretch for my next goal.

- Going deeper into my community is important for my success.

- I'm learning how to be better in the 'non-exercise parts' of my life.

- I am always looking for ways to evolve my goal-setting process.

- Using the tools and strategies I have learnt to this point in time is a wise thing to do.

Workbook for Baby Step 7

Before you start doing this workbook go back and read your post-event reflection work. This will help you see where you need to grow and what you need to reinforce around what you do well.

Here are the questions for this workbook:

1. How can I evolve my goal-setting process?

2. Who do I need to work with in setting this goal and what questions do I have for them?

3. How can I use my goal-setting processes to set myself up for success?

4. When is the best time for me to do my goal-setting session?

5. Based on a development pathway, what is the wisest stretch goal for my exercise journey?

6. Is this goal realistic for the time I have to commit to exercise?

7. How will this help me develop myself as an exerciser?

8. How can I get more aligned and involved with my community?

9. What are some personal areas I can develop (like planning) through achieving this goal?

10. Why is it important for me to set my next fitness goal so quickly and what will be the benefits of me doing this?

Where to from here?

From here you will move towards achieving your second fitness goal. The aim at the end will be another completed goal but also for you to learn and evolve towards having fitness in your life. You will learn more and more about how to become a long-term exerciser and how to be a higher version of yourself.

The journey of this book divides now because while you are moving towards achieving your second fitness goal the lessons in the next few Baby Steps are about cementing exercise for the long term, so you become that lifetime lover of exercise.

As soon as you have completed the work for this step you can move onto the next Baby Steps. You'll be able to implement these Baby Steps as you are achieving this goal. Be excited because you are able to go to a place that will completely change how you see yourself and the future you are going to experience.

Success in this step equals:

- You will have set your second fitness goal two weeks after your first goal achievement.

- You will have the perfect stretch goal in place, based on your development pathway.

- You will have found ways, and committed to, being more involved with your community.

- You will have started the work of achieving your next fitness goal.

- You will have evolved your processes around goal setting.

Imagine...

You now have your second fitness goal in place. A goal that is realistic, allows you to grown in the wisest way possible and one that you are excited to move towards. Having this next challenge will keep you motivated and connected to your movement and the people who are helping you with your exercise journey. Having this second goal means you are cementing fitness in your life for the long term. You have experienced this once before—now go and get it!

Share your Second Goal

Once you have set your second goal to to our social page and share it.
Use hashtag #mysecondgoal

To join our social pages go to:
www.passionaboutexercise.com/social

Remember you can sign up for the Passion for Exercise course by going to:
www.passionaboutexercise.com/course

Chapter 10

When you see yourself this way you will love exercise forever

I was in Sweden for one of the biggest fitness workshops I had ever presented at. The class I was taking had over 2,000 people in it. It was one of those moments in life where the experience actually exceeded the expectation. Imagine walking on stage to a couple of thousand people that are excited to see you there and can't wait to have an amazing fitness experience. I had goosebumps as I went on stage. This was definitely a career highlight for me.

I've been lucky in my fitness career to have a few of these 'big moment' highlights, where I've travelled around the world and taught massive fitness classes to people who were passionate about the workout we would be doing together. While I've loved all of these experiences, often these trips have other benefits, benefits that actually exceed the 'big moment' highlights.

Back to Sweden. The day before I was going to be doing my presentation I went down for breakfast at the hotel restaurant. I'm always up early which means when I travel I'm often the first person in the restaurant. Sometimes I'll have the whole place to myself. This was one of those mornings as when I walked in at

6am there was no one else in the room.

As I went to the buffet I turned around to see that Jackie Mills had entered the room. Jackie Mills is a fitness legend. She is one of the key figures in the world-leading fitness brand Les Mills. For years she has been a leader who has had a massive influence on the direction and trends of the fitness industry. Jackie is one of those people who has an aura of wisdom, her knowledge and understanding is of the highest level in all areas of life but it's the next level when it comes to fitness.

Luckily for me I've known Jackie for years but because we live in different cities I have had limited time with her. She's one of those people that makes you feel you can do more with your life. She has an ability to help you see possibility within yourself and can help to guide you to your next level, so any time you get to spend quality time with her you jump at the opportunity.

As I was getting the last bit of my breakfast Jackie came up to me and asked if I wanted to have breakfast together. This was one of those opportunities—I jumped at it.

The thing about wise people is that they often have a curiosity about them. Of course they have a lot to offer but they often seem more intrigued by what they can learn from others. This is Jackie to a tee. As we sat down Jackie started asking me questions about my life. These questions were the type of questions that opened you up to deeper conversations. Because Jackie creates a trusting environment you find yourself showing all of who you are.

After talking about life Jackie asked me about my business. I had briefly told her about it in the past so she had a general idea of what we did but she was interested to know about our beginner 5km group and the lessons that I had learnt in putting my focus on helping beginners. Again, Jackie showed her wisdom. She had so much knowledge with fitness but she was trying to learn from me in an area that I had experienced success in.

I went on to share some of the key insights I had learnt since I had started my beginner group. Jackie seemed to be absorbing every word I was telling her, she was like a reporter coming back to me with questions that helped to gain a deeper understanding of what I was sharing. She was making me feel like I was the teacher and she was the student.

After a bit of time Jackie asked me a question that I hadn't spent much time thinking about before this moment. She asked me when I thought these people go from being non-exercisers to being people who know that they will have exercise in their life for the long term.

This created a need for me to pause. Up until this moment I hadn't really thought about this. I knew we were doing a great job with helping people start their running journey by getting them to run 5km and that many of our people would go on to complete half marathons with us, but when did that switch happen, that moment where they transitioned into a long-term exerciser, I hadn't thought about this.

Then the answer appeared in my head. There's always a moment that I experience with our runners who have started from nothing and go on to do a half marathon. They come up to me in a way that shows me they are proud of themselves and say that when they see other runners now they feel like they are one of them. When you look at other runners and feel like you are one of them that means you have the behaviours that this group of people have, it means you have an understanding of what it means to be this person, it means you feel a belonging and ownership of the identity of a runner. The other side of this is that when you are missing your running training you feel you are losing yourself, you feel dissonance because you are the type of person who runs, so when you aren't it feels wrong. My job is to get people to the point where they have a sense of identity with movement in their life. It's not something they know they should do, it's something they do because it's a part of who they are.

My conversation with Jackie helped me identify the place I was trying to get people to with exercise. When I think about myself, I see myself as a healthy and fit man and because I have this self identity there are actions and behaviours that I prioritise in my life. This self-identity means that I don't buy fast food, that I'll aim to exercise six days a week, that I make sure I get good sleep and have healthy relationships in my life. When I'm not doing these things I feel like I'm losing myself, it feels wrong and I want to get back to those actions and behaviours asap.

I like to think of my identity as something I work to reinforce. When I have experiences that reinforce my identity I tell myself, 'This is proof that I'm a fit and healthy person'. This is also why people with strong identities around health and fitness feel a disconnect when they are falling away from exercise or healthy habits. They feel like they are losing themselves because this isn't who they are. This dissonance is a good thing because it motivates them to get back to their healthy habits.

This is the place we are trying to get you to in this book. I want you to have an inner-identity that is based around exercise and a healthy lifestyle. I want you to get to the place where when you aren't doing your exercise you feel like you are losing yourself, which means you'll be motivated to get back to it asap. That's why we have our next Baby Step:

Baby Step 8: Take ownership of your fitness identity so it becomes a part of how you see yourself

If you are at this stage of your journey in this book you have made a huge amount of positive change in your life, including:

- You have learnt how to prioritise putting exercise in your life.
- You have found a movement you enjoy.
- You have found your community.
- You have developed your fitness and skills.
- You have achieved a fitness goal.
- You have learnt how to function at higher levels in all areas of your life.

All of that change is massive but we haven't even mentioned the more tangible benefits you have experienced. I imagine these may include:

- You have more energy.

- You are fitter.

- You may have lost weight and are leaner.

- You have better self-esteem.

- You have opened yourself up to other possibilities in your life.

- You have improved confidence.

- You have developed positive relationships.

- You feel better about your life.

Stop and reread that list, those are huge!!!

If you are at this point you are no longer the person who started this journey. Think back to the way you saw yourself with exercise before this started. I imagine your inner dialog would have probably looked something like this:

- I'm not an exerciser.

- I don't like... (insert a type of exercise here, like running).

- I just don't have time to exercise.

- I can't exercise because I get injured.

- I know I should exercise but other things are more important.

- Exercise is just too hard.

You may recognise these statements from the old version of you and you may still hold on to some of these, or ones like these, but your job now is to take ownership of the new you. We want you to 100% self-identify as being an exerciser.

This isn't a 'fake it till you make it' thing. This is about you using the evidence of your experience to reinforce who you now are, and to consciously keep reinforcing it so you 100% feel this identity is you. By doing this you will be that person who exercises because that's who you are, and you will feel you are losing yourself when you fall away from exercise. Once you have arrived at this point you'll have exercise for the long term.

Challenge for Baby Step 8

To create a routine that uses your exercise experiences to build evidence that reinforces your identity as an exerciser.

Rules for Baby Step 8

RULE #1: Make a commitment to a conscious process that catches and gives you ownership of the evidence around your fitness identity

If you want to improve your life one of the easiest ways to do this is with a gratitude process. Martin Seligman, one of the leaders in positive psychology, covers this in his book *Flourish*. He talks about how studies show that a gratitude process is proven to improve your life and this process can be as simple as spending ten minutes every night identifying three things that have happened that day that you are grateful for and why they happened. For example, a friend may have bought you an ice cream on a hot day and this happened because you are a good person in your friend's life, so they wanted to do something nice for you.

I think we can all understand that having a gratitude process like this is worth doing. I can pretty much guarantee that you have heard of this or something like this before but the problem is, most people don't do it. So many people want to improve their life but they don't commit to the strategies that work, even simple ones that only take ten minutes.

For strategies to work we have to commit to doing them and ideally we want to make them part of our daily routine. For example I write in a journal every night, I write about my day and at the end of this I always finish with what I learnt, what I gave and three good things from my day. Because I have attached this process to a nightly habit it is now part of my daily routine.

When we get to the strategies section for this Baby Step I'm going to offer some that will build your self identity around fitness. Don't just think, 'That's a good idea, I should try that'. Commit to a regular time where you will apply the technique. Aim to make it a routine that you do at a regular time so it just becomes a way of life for you. This commitment will fast-forward your ownership of you being an exerciser which is important to your long-term exercising self.

RULE #2: No 'Yes, buts'

Have you heard of a 'Yes, but'? It may not seem obvious but there's a chance that you have used it in your life more than once or twice.

A 'Yes, but' is when you do well at something but you diminish it by not giving yourself the credit you deserve. It's the person who is on a 20kg weight loss journey, has worked hard and created some amazing changes to get themselves half way there by losing 10kg. Instead of owning their success up to this point they tell themselves, 'Yes, but you are still overweight'. Or it's the person who has gotten back into exercise and has just achieved the goal of doing a 40km mountain bike race but they tell themselves, 'Yes, but you were at the back of the field.'

Not only does a 'Yes, but' diminish your success and take away good feelings you should be owning, it lessens your ability to take ownership of the character traits that maintain your growth and build your identity in the areas you are being successful in.

Let's go back to the 20kg weight loss example. The person has done amazingly well to lose 10kg and there will be many behavioural and identity shifts that they should be taking ownership of, for example the self-talk they should be using is:

- I'm good at planning my food.

- I know how to manage my emotions so I don't look to food during stressful times.

- I know how to include basic movement into my life.

- I know how to choose healthy foods.

You can see that if someone has ownership of these self-identity statements it becomes easier to lose the last 10kg of their weight loss journey. When you inject a 'Yes, but' into the experience you are focusing on why you aren't there and why you will probably fail.

A 'Yes, but' says:

- I've been good at planning my food but every time in the past I have fallen off the wagon.

- I know how to manage my emotions but I haven't had a really stressful situation where I'll look to food for comfort.

- I know how to put basic movement in my life but when I get busy I'll probably end up quitting.

- I know how to choose healthy foods but I always end up giving in to junk food eventually.

In some ways it makes sense why people have their 'Yes, buts'— they don't trust themselves. Sure they have done well to this point but their history may show them that they have gone back to square one in the past. It's like the 'Yes, but' is a safety net, it gives you an out if you do fail. If you do go back to where you started, you can say, 'I knew this would happen'.

We want you to build trust and confidence in your ability. The 'Yes, but' undermines your trust and confidence. We want you to be the person who can 100% believe the identity that creates long term success. We want you to be able to know within yourself that:

- I'm the type of person who knows how to have exercise in my life.

- I am fit and healthy.

- I enjoy being active.

- I can take on a challenge.

When you 100% believe this and feel these things are just a part of who you are you'll have exercise in your life forever. Don't let your 'Yes, buts' work against you instilling your exercise identity.

Dealing with the 'Yes, buts'

There's a simple process you can use to help you deal with your Yes, buts, it goes like this:

1. Catch yourself when you are using your Yes, buts

This is about creating an awareness of when you are doing this and aim to become a master of catching yourself before you use a 'Yes, but' statement. It could be when you are talking to other people or it could be within your own inner-dialogue.

2. Tell yourself that your 'Yes, buts' don't serve you in any way

This is about reminding yourself that your 'Yes, buts' are working against you, that they offer no value and you don't need to believe them.

3. Use an alignment/evidence statement

There's a good technique called 'I am... because... which means ...'. I like to call it an alignment/evidence statement.

For example, 'I am good at planning my food because for the last week I got up every morning and planned my food for that day. This means that I can trust that I can continue doing this for the next week.'

The above statement uses evidence to reinforce the alignment of your identity. You are good at planning your food, you have

197

done that well which is proof that you can continue on the path you are on.

4. Look to take more actions that reinforce your identity

Look to the next moment where you can build evidence that will reinforce the identity that is good for you. Once you find it, predetermine the actions that you will take. In the food planning example you can see that you will get up early tomorrow and you will do your food planning again.

By removing your 'Yes, buts' you are massively increasing your ability to take ownership of your growth. It may take some time but the better you get at practising these techniques the faster it will happen.

Strategies for Baby Step 8

STRATEGY #1: Use proof and 'Ownership Statements' after every reinforcing experience

As I said before my neighbours must think I'm a bit weird. Every so often they will see me running towards my driveway and see me pumping my arms in the air like I've just won the Olympic marathon. It does look a bit odd but there's a good reason why it happens.

I have this rule that when I have an amazing run, where I work really hard and challenge myself, when I see my driveway at the end of the run I pick up my speed to a sprint and then pump my arms in the air like I have won a race. This is me catching a moment I can be proud of and having a little emotionally-charged celebration to myself. Inside my head I tell myself, 'This is proof that I'm good at pushing myself hard'.

I want to reinforce the good moments in my training and I want to reinforce character traits that are important to me. If I didn't do my self celebration I would still know that I've had a good run but this process deepens the good feelings and reinforces personal character traits to a deeper level.

This is an example of capturing the things we want to reinforce in the moment we experience them, it's something I want you to practise within this Baby Step. There's a really simple three-step technique that you can use to do this:

1. Spend some time identifying the identity, character traits, and habits that you want to be aligned with

You might write them down as Ownership Statements that you hold around your identity, character traits, and habits around your health and fitness and these may include:

- I'm a consistent exerciser.

- I'm good at planning exercise in my life.

- I'm someone who can stick to a programme.

- I enjoy having exercise in my life.

2. Catch when you have experiences that reinforce your identity, character traits, and habits

You have a session with your training group that is a lot of fun, you have heaps of laughs and while you have completed your exercise for the day it seemed easy because of how fun it was. This experience is an example of you enjoying having exercise in your life.

Or you have managed to complete every session your programme had for you this week. This is an example that you are someone who can stick to a programme.

Remember, no 'Yes, buts' here.

3. Attach your Ownership Statement to the experience

Once you have evidence, use an Ownership Statement. You could say, 'This is proof that I enjoy exercise' or 'This is an example of me being someone who can stick to a programme'.

It's as simple as this. Because you have identified the identity, character traits, and habits you want you can capture the moments where you are actually experiencing these and stamp your Ownership Statement on top of them.

At first you may not 100% feel ownership of your statements but the more you attach them to real experiences the more evidence you are creating that you are that person. After a while you won't need to consciously inject these in; you'll find that when you have the experience your mind will subconsciously do this for you.

STRATEGY #2: Talk about yourself in your new identity

Here's a fun experiment to try the next time you are at a party or another social setting where people are talking in a group, especially if you don't know the people very well. Spend time being the ultimate listener and see how much you can learn about each person in the group as individuals. It's amazing how much you can learn about people if you just put your listening and learning cap on.

In social settings a lot of conversation can be about who we are as people. Someone will say, 'I love to travel' and then someone else will agree and this will trigger a flow of conversation. Someone else may say, 'Travelling is not my thing, I'm more into tramping'.

Those statements are activity statements but then there are the identity statements that we use such as, 'I'm not the most organised person', 'I'm a caring person', 'I'm a good problem solver' or conversely, negative statements like, 'I'm no good with willpower', 'I'm easily frustrated', 'I don't like exercise'. These statements reveal a deeper level of a person.

You can learn a lot about people just by sitting and listening. We reveal so much about ourselves. Where it gets interesting is to think about how you reveal yourself to your world. When you are in situations where you are sharing the kind of person you are, both with activity statements and identity statements what do you say?

If you break this down into different areas of your life what do you say? For example, what do you say about yourself around:

- your career

- your relationships

- your eating habits

- your exercise habits

- how you deal with tough times

- the things you love doing

A part of you shifting and taking ownership of your exercising self is for you to start expressing and communicating the new version of yourself to the world. This may be really hard at first and there are a few reasons for this. While your experiences are evidence and proof that you are this new person it may not 100% sit comfortably with you just yet so you hold back on expressing it. Or, you may feel that you have so much progress to make and you are worried about judgement from others if you say that you are good at exercise. I completely understand these mindsets but they restrict you from taking full ownership and will prolong the process.

If you do feel uncomfortable about changing your communication about yourself, spend some time identifying how you can express yourself in a way that you are comfortable with. To do this use the Step Back approach. This is where you start with your ultimate statement (that you may at first feel uncomfortable using). Let's say it's: 'I'm a regular exerciser who has a great routine'.

You may feel like you will be judged if you use this statement as you still feel you are a little overweight and therefore not quite identifying with this statement 100% so expressing this is hard. Using the Step Back approach is to go back a few steps with this statement and say: 'I'm in the process of developing a regular exercise routine and I'm finding that I'm being consistent with it. I'm really enjoying it'.

You can see that this approach allows you to have ownership of the new you but it's a bit safer. When you use the Step Back approach you are taking it back to a level that you are comfortable with. If this statement still feels uncomfortable, take it back another step: 'I've started exercising with the aim of learning how to have a consistent routine'.

Keep taking steps back until you find the place where you are comfortable expressing your ownership. As time goes on you want to move up the levels and become comfortable with your ultimate statement and while you will get there, the Step Back approach allows you to safely shift away from the old version of yourself more gradually.

Once you have identified how you can comfortably express the newer version of yourself, you want to catch moments where you will communicate this with your world. At first you need to be quite conscious about this as you are shifting from a historic pattern. See the moments where you are talking about health and fitness and then practise your new statements. It may feel weird at first but the more you do it the easier it will become. Notice what happens. You'll probably find that you aren't rejected and that most people just want to talk about themselves anyway, or they may be curious about your experiences and ask you questions.

This is an important strategy because the more you can express yourself outwardly to your world the more you cement the 'exercising you' inside yourself. The thing to always remember is that you are not a fraud—this identity is based on the evidence you have built over the last period of your life. You are this person, it's ok for you to express it. Actually, it's wise for you to express it.

STRATEGY #3: Align more deeply with your tribe by expanding outside of your community

By now in your journey you will have a deep understanding of why community is so important to your exercise success. You will have developed friendships, had shared experiences, felt higher levels of motivation, had fun, and experienced belonging. To me, finding your community is the number one key to success in a fitness journey.

In this Baby Step we are looking to deepen your connection with your exercising world. It's about feeling alignment to the bigger world of your movement.

Back when I was doing Ironman I managed to qualify for the Hawaii Ironman. Achieving a finish in an Ironman is a massive goal but getting to the Hawaii Ironman is another level because you have to qualify for it. This means you have to be the next-level athlete. During race week at the Hawaii Ironman you walk down the street and you are surrounded by some of the fittest people in the world.

I remember the day before I was racing, I was talking to a guy in the race registration line. He said to me that only around 30,000 people in the history of the world have ever done this race and that I'll be joining a special group of people when I cross the finish line tomorrow. His comment was powerful, it hit me in a big way and it made me feel a connection to something bigger. I was a part of the worldwide Ironman community and I was proud to be one of these people.

Experiencing alignment with your tribe, outside of your community can be done in many ways, such as:

- being a passionate follower of the elite level of your sport

- seeking out the content of the higher-level leaders of your sport through listening to a podcast or watching some YouTube clips

- becoming a fan of a team or certain athletes

- reading books on the sport

- buying the clothing brands that your tribe wears

- participating in activities that your tribe takes part in

The more you absorb yourself in your movement the more you will feel that sense of alignment to your tribe. This attachment becomes part of your identity which will keep you in your activity.

STRATEGY #4: Live and maintain the standards of your tribe

The other day I was on the phone to a friend of mine, one of the world's top fitness instructors, Lisa Osborne. Lisa is a megastar in the fitness world. She has achieved everything in fitness, from being a world champion in her sport to being one of the most recognised faces in the fitness industry. I feel lucky to have worked beside Lisa in my career as I have learnt so much from her and she has always had a strong sense of what is important in creating successful fitness experiences for people.

I was having a chat with Lisa on the phone about this book and the step that I'm writing right now. Because I had a guru on the line I thought I would ask her what she felt was the key to creating ownership of a fitness identity. Lisa instantly started talking about respecting and maintaining the standards of your tribe. She talked about how when she's training she wants to make sure she's living up to the standards of the people who are at the highest level in her tribe and wants to help others experience this level as well. This was such a great insight and it made me think of an example I have of this from my life.

One of the biggest tribes I have been part of is the Les Mills instructor tribe. Les Mills has thousands of instructors around the world and we are a very passionate bunch. When people become Les Mills instructors they experience one of the most rewarding times in their lives because they are challenged to grow in so many different ways in such a short period of time.

Becoming an instructor means you need to be fit, you need to develop your ability to teach fitness in front of groups of people, you have to learn how to motivate people, and you have to learn hundreds of skills that create a fitness experience that people want to come to. It's hard to become an instructor but the growth you experience is phenomenal and the rewards of being an instructor make it all worth it.

When people first start out as an instructor they do everything it takes to do a good job, partly because they know what they need to do to develop themselves but also because they are so passionate. Sadly, for some instructors, after a period of time they stop growing and lose the passion they once had at the beginning of their career. These instructors know how to do the job well but they have lost the love. I call these people the 'old school instructors'. They are using the tools of the trade from when they started. It can be as simple as the music they use down to how they motivate their people. It's the same old same old, they often haven't evolved in a long time.

I remember when I first started instructing at my gym there was an instructor like this. He took a good class but you could tell that he had let his standards drop. His classes were always the same, the music was the same, his language was the same, his gear looked ten years old and I remember thinking to myself, 'I never want to become that guy' and I can proudly say that I haven't.

I've been teaching since 1999 and to this day I'm still as passionate as I was at the beginning of my journey. The reason I still have this passion is that I've always maintained high standards, the high standards that the best in my game also maintain which include:

- Always be current with the trends, education and workouts.

- Always turn up prepared.

- Keep my physical self at a role-model level.

- Do the 'behind the scenes' work that keeps me sharp.

- Always respect that people are letting me lead them so lead them in a way that helps them grow.

It's through maintaining these standards that has helped me continually grow at an activity that I have been doing for a very long time. It has kept me at a high level and has kept my passion alive. It's also rewarding because it helps me be a role model for younger instructors as they don't see me as an 'old school instructor'. They see that they can have a career where the passion and growth can continue for a long time.

For you to deepen the ownership of your fitness identity you want to start to create an understanding of the standards you want to maintain, but you also want to understand the standards that the higher-level people in your world work to. Once you gain an insight into these you can start to aim to live up to these standards.

A good practical step to take at this stage is to identify two different types of standards: the current standards you should aim to maintain and the aspirational standards that you can look to aim for. Your current standards represent where you currently are with your exercise, while the aspirational standards would be the ones the higher-level people in your movement hold.

Once you have identified with these you will have a baseline that you don't want to drop below and a vision of where you can go in the future.

STRATEGY #5: Aim to achieve the landmark goals of your tribe

Running is a great example. The total beginner is over the moon when they achieve the goal of running 5km, the next goal then becomes to run 10km, after that there's the half marathon, and then there's the massive goal of running a marathon. Many runners use these same stepping stone goals or what I like to call 'landmark goals'.

There are other landmark goals for a runner such as doing one of the popular 'big city marathons' like the New York Marathon. This is a 'bucket list' marathon for many runners so much so they have to reject nearly 50,000 applications for the race each year, and this is a race with over 50,000 competitors!

Most activities will have their own landmark goals and by aiming to achieve these you get that sense of belonging to a bigger world which deepens the roots of your fitness identity.

STRATEGY #6: Share your experience with your world

A good way to reinforce your fitness identity is to share it. I totally understand that when people first start their fitness journey they can feel vulnerable and insecure, they can doubt that they will be successful and for this reason they protect themselves by not telling anyone what they are doing.

I was talking to one of our new runners the other day and she said no one knew she was doing this and they wouldn't know unless she ran 5km. I didn't push back on this because this allowed her to feel safe and it was what she needed to do at this stage in her journey. But if you have got to this stage in the book and have achieved a couple of fitness goals of your own this may be a good time to share some of your experiences with your world.

When it comes to sharing your experiences you have to do it in a way that feels right to you. My lovely wife Jo is more of a private person than I am. She'll share that she's aiming for a goal but it will only be with close friends and family, whereas I would share the experience with my entire world. The thing to remember here is that there is no wrong or right way of sharing your experience, it's about sharing it in a way that's right for you.

One of the benefits of sharing your experiences with your world is it shifts how your world sees you. I remember when I was competing in Ironman triathlons the first question anyone would ask me when I started a conversation with them was 'how's training going?'. This was because my world understood that I was an athlete and that I loved exercising. By sharing your experiences, your world will see you in a new light—another reinforcement of your fitness identity.

STRATEGY #7: Learn to identify dissonance and realise this is a good thing

When we have a strong identity in one area, if we do something that goes against what this identity represents we feel a sense of dissonance. It could be that you pride yourself on never being a gossip and you live by the theory of 'If I don't have something good to say I won't say anything at all'. If you then find yourself in a social setting where you are talking about others and you say something negative or you spread some gossip, you feel that you have done something wrong. It's this dissonance that's reminding you that you aren't a gossip and you don't like that you have done this.

Lifetime lovers of exercise feel this way when they are out of their exercise routine. Let's say you like to do five training sessions a week where you mix up some strength, skill, and cardio work. When you are in a routine you feel aligned and that you are being true to yourself but then work gets a bit crazy and suddenly you are time-poor which means your exercise routine stops. You might go a day or two when you can justify this place but the longer you leave it the more dissonance you feel. You feel like you are losing yourself because you aren't doing something that is important to you and is aligned to your identity.

Understanding dissonance at this stage in your journey is important. Firstly, because it's amazing that you have it, if you have dissonance because you aren't exercising that means that you've instilled the fitness identity within yourself and it feels wrong for you not to exercise. Be proud that you have this feeling, it's one of the keys to becoming a lifetime lover of exercise.

Secondly, when you feel dissonance you want to use it as a guide to motivate you to get back to your exercise routine. The faster you feel and catch dissonance the faster you can get back on track. When you feel dissonance, remind yourself that it's your job to get back to the version of yourself where you feel aligned to your fitness identity and use good strategies and planning to make this happen.

STRATEGY #8: See the value of your shift

Earlier in this step I identified all of the amazing benefits you will have experienced throughout this journey—the fitness, the personal growth, the connections and experiences you have had and so on. One of the best ways to take ownership of your fitness self is to see and fully embrace the shifts you have made. They have created a new you so as you experience these shifts see the value they bring to your life.

Notice how your life is different because you have more energy, that you have deep connections with your tribe, that you can achieve goals, and that you feel better about yourself. By seeing the value of your shifts it makes it more attractive for you to stay on the path you're on and it makes it easier for you to reinforce your fitness identity.

STRATEGY #9: Learn about yourself

While I have offered strategies that will help you to see yourself as an exerciser you also want to see the opportunities for you to deepen this. It's like you have a beacon within yourself that is there to catch and see the moments that reinforce this identity.

It might be a work colleague asking about how you got into exercise or noticing that you can get out the door and go for a run without even thinking about it (something the old version of you could never have contemplated). There will be many small moments that will give you the opportunity to keep reinforcing your fitness identity. Be like a sponge with these, soak them up and stamp them to the identity of you being an exerciser.

Mindsets to practise for Baby Step 8

- It's my job to take ownership of my fitness identity.

- When I hear myself saying 'Yes', but I will stop myself and allow myself to own my growth.

- I will become a beacon for catching moments that reinforce my identity.

- It's good for me to share my fitness experiences.

- I will have the courage to talk about my exercising self.

- The deeper I can engage with my tribe the better.

- I will hold the standards of my tribe high.
- It's good to express myself as an exerciser.

Workbook for Baby Step 8

Baby Step 8's workbook is designed to help you to 100% own your fitness identity. Work through these questions and put your answers into practice in your everyday life.

1. What is my Ownership Statement for my fitness? (Remember to use the Step Back approach if you are struggling).
2. How will I represent myself around health and fitness to my world?
3. How can I become great at catching evidence of my new fitness self and what will I do when I catch these moments?
4. How will I catch my 'Yes, buts' and where will I put my focus?
5. What can I do to deeply align myself with my fitness community? (Think learning, books, people to follow on social media, gear).
6. What are the standards of my tribe? Where do I sit within these right now and where can I develop myself to evolve my standards?
7. What are the landmark goals of my tribe? Of these, what are the realistic ones at this stage of my journey?
8. What's the best way for me to share my shift with my world?
9. How can I become better at seeing the benefits of my shift?
10. What else can I do to reinforce my fitness identity?

Where to from here?

This step is so important because it leads to a shift in how you see yourself. Once this shift is in place your exercise habit will become easier, because that's what someone like you does.

When we think about the journey of this book you can get the work done for this step while you are achieving your second fitness goal. If this is where you are at right now, hold off on moving to Baby Step 9 until your second goal is complete.

If you have completed your second fitness goal you can move onto Baby Step 9 now.

Success in this Step equals:

- You will have done the work in the workbook.

- You will have an understanding of your new identity and will be using the tools and strategies in this step to reinforce this.

- You will be taking actions that deepen your connection to your tribe.

- The way you express yourself to your world will be as someone who is an exerciser.

- When you are missing exercise you will feel dissonance which you will use to get you back on track.

- You'll be using your exercise experiences to build evidence of your new identity.

- You'll see yourself as an exerciser.

Imagine...

Imagine if you 100% identified with yourself as an exerciser, that you felt aligned to your tribe and were happy to express your fitness identity to your world. Imagine feeling regret if you miss your exercise session which in turn motivates you to get back on track. How would your life be better if you were in this place?

This can be you. Follow these steps and it won't be far away.

Share how you are changing how you see yourself

As you build evidence of you shifting and how you see yourself, go on our social pages and share it with us. Make sure you add the hashtag #newme

To join our social pages go to:
www.passionaboutexercise.com/social

Remember you can sign up for the Passion for Exercise course by going to:
www.passionaboutexercise.com/course

Chapter 11

The tool that will help you thrive with exercise for the long term

Years ago I wrote my first book with my friend Fraser. Don't bother searching for it because it never got past the first draft! The motivation for the book was a concept that I called the 'Circle of Fitness'. Actually, the real motivation was to create a solution to a curiosity I had.

Working in fitness you see different types of people. There are the ones you never see (people who never exercise); the ones who have a one-off moment where fitness is in their lives and then it disappears; the yo-yo person who comes and goes from fitness; the person who has a fitness habit but never creates any change; and then you have the person who consistently thrives with fitness, gets amazing results and experiences the benefits for the long term.

When we look at the person who is thriving with fitness we see someone who tends to have an inner trust. These people know that they will exercise their whole life, they understand what it takes to not only keep the habit of exercise up, they know how to do it in ways that get them the best results so they enjoy the benefits for the long term.

My curiosity led me to this question: 'What do people who thrive with fitness have and what can they teach to others so we can get more people thriving with fitness for the long term?'. With this question in mind I approached one of my best mates, Fraser, to see if he wanted to write a book with me that tried to answer this question.

At that time I was really into the self-help guru, Og Mandino. It's funny looking back on my commitment to Og's books. He had a book called *The Greatest Salesman in the World* which was directed at salespeople but it was really about strengthening character so you wouldn't quit. The books were written like a biblical tale where the main character had to learn lessons about what it took to be successful. These lessons included 'I will persist until I succeed', 'Never feel shame for trying and failing for he who has never failed is he who has never tried', and 'I will form good habits and become their slave'.

At the end of each step he had created a long-form affirmation based on the lessons learnt from that step, and these affirmations took five to ten minutes to read. Og's suggestion was for you to spend a month reading the same affirmation every morning, once you had completed that month you went on to the next affirmation in the book.

Because I was a dedicated student I was committed to his formula. Every morning for the next year I got up and read one of his long-form affirmations. While Og's work seems a bit dated these days I still have moments in my life where my inner voice tells me 'I will persist till I succeed'.

With Og's influence in place my mate Fraser and I sat down to write our book. The concept we developed was the Circle of Fitness and like Og's books it was told like a historic tale of a person being mentored by a wise soul through the Circle of Fitness journey.

After spending a couple of months together writing I gave the first draft to a book critic I knew from my local newspaper and one thing I can tell you about this critic, she was honest. Her feedback was that our book was like an extreme religious rhetoric and she felt that we were probably best to go back to the drawing board with our approach on how to write it.

As honest and harsh as her feedback was, she did say to make sure we do start again because while the way we have written it doesn't work, the Circle of Fitness is a great idea that a lot of people would learn a lot from.

Feeling despondent, the project fell away, life moved on and that book became a distant memory.

That was until I sat down to design the Baby Steps for this book. I knew this book was about helping people through the first stages of their fitness journey but the real aim was to create a lifetime love of fitness, a place where people can trust that they will always have exercise in their lives and they will thrive.

This is where the Circle of Fitness comes in. It's a mindset/strategy that will not only help you have exercise in your life for the long term, it will help you thrive with exercise for the rest of your life.

So let's look at the next Baby Step.

Baby Step 9: Develop the ability to live within the Circle of Fitness for the long term

The Circle of Fitness is a model that you move through and can be repeated over and over again. It allows you to challenge yourself, continue to get results and evolve what fitness means in your life.

Here's how it works:

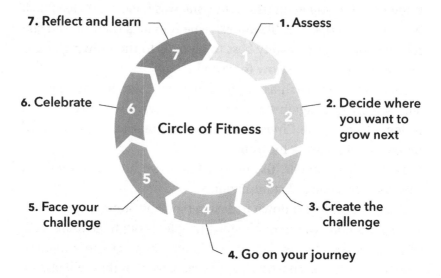

Let's break down the steps:

1. Assess

When you get to the beginning of each circle phase in your fitness life do an assessment of where you currently are. This will ask questions about where you are physically, mentally, where you are within the activity you enjoy, and any other area that you feel is important to your exercise life (which could include things like the social side of exercise). This step is all about painting a clear picture of the actual place you are in *right now*.

The aim is to be as accurate as possible at this stage. The more honest and factual you can be, the better. You'll then be able to progress to the next step.

2. Decide where you want to grow next

Once you have done your assessment and you have a clear picture of your current self, determine where you want to grow within your health and fitness over the next period of time.

Through having a clear understanding of your current self you will be able to make wise decisions about your next steps. For example, you may know you have a busy time ahead within your career so how you can grow with your health and fitness will need to be realistic based on your time limitations.

The good thing about this step is there are so many ways you can grow. Your growth could be a special skill you feel you need to develop within your movement, it could be a mental toughness challenge, it could be to be more engaged with the social side of your movement, it could even be to become a more organised person so you train more effectively.

The growth you are looking for is about aiming to evolve yourself in both your movement and as a person.

3. Create the challenge

Now that you have a good understanding of where you currently are with your health and fitness and you know where you want to grow, you can set a challenge that fits within your life and will evolve you at the same time.

The aim here is to find the perfect challenge for you right now which you can realistically achieve within the constraints of your life. By getting this right you will feel excited because you have found the right goal to work towards.

4. Go on your journey

Now you are going to pull your socks up, get out there and do the work of getting ready to achieve the challenge. The journey will include planning (like you do in your goal-setting process), doing the work (like your training and skill development), getting support and advice from your mentors, and so on.

5. Face your challenge

This is your testing moment, the moment you have worked towards in Baby Step 4. Challenges are so good for you because they give you the opportunity to go to places you have never been before.

Although your challenge may be focussed on performance, it's also about your inner experience. You may feel nervous and doubtful because you are stretching yourself, but this is a great place to be as it shows you that you are aiming to grow and extend yourself.

6. Celebrate

After any challenge you want to devote some time to celebrating, even if you didn't get the full outcome you desired. The celebration needs to cover the whole training period, from the moment you created the challenge. Your celebration needs to be in a way that feels right to you.

7. Reflect and Learn

Look back on the last period of time and see what lessons you can learn. This should cover all aspects of your journey. You can reinforce what you did well and identify some areas that you can work on moving forward. This is a powerful step because it will help you identify where you can set your sights as you head towards a new round of the Circle of Fitness.

Once you've done one loop of the Circle of Fitness you go back to square one. Because you have evolved over the last period you will have new areas to grow in, you'll find new challenges, and you'll set off on a new adventure.

You can see that if you're committed to following this process you will become that person that thrives with fitness in the long term and is constantly evolving. It's exciting when you think about it.

Challenge for Baby Step 9

To set up a life where you have a commitment to the Circle of Fitness for the long term.

Rules for Baby Step 9

RULE #1: Commit to the process for the next 12 months

If you have followed the steps in this book and applied them to your life I imagine you have created massive change and there are many benefits you will have experienced. You will have also learnt some valuable lessons. One of these lessons is that if you want to change you have to put effort into the processes that will create change.

The last thing I want to happen is for you to take a step backwards and fall back to where you were before you started this book. My aim has always been for you to *create a lifetime love of fitness.*

By focusing on taking all of the lessons in this book and committing the effort to go through the steps of the Circle of Fitness for the next year you are cementing exercise in your life, for the long term.

Make this your goal for the next 12 months and you are locking in a healthier future.

Strategies for Baby Step 9

STRATEGY #1: Use all the lessons that you have learnt so far

I once interviewed a world-leading educational expert. He gave me what I thought was the best definition of education: Education is the ability to truly teach people how to understand something they didn't know and for them to be able to apply this knowledge in the world.

I loved this definition because it was so obvious but clearly correct! What's the point in cramming for a test if you don't truly understand what you have learnt and can't apply your learnings and understandings?

The experience you have been through with this book as your guide will have taught you so many valuable lessons. You will have a new understanding about having exercise in your life and you want to move forward and apply the lessons you have learnt and use them in the wisest way possible. You may even want to spend time writing down what you have learnt and how you can apply this in your next stage.

STRATEGY #2: Keep using your tribe/community

I know I'm beating the same drum here so I'll keep it short. Get your people involved with your experience within the Circle of Fitness.

STRATEGY #3: Catch if you are falling away from the Circle of Fitness

Going back to the different types of exercisers I described earlier in this step, the one I find most interesting is the one who has the habit but never creates any change. Don't get me wrong, I think that you are much better off to be in this place than being a yo-yo person or not doing any exercise at all but the 'habit' people are missing out on so much that could be quickly shifted if they used the Circle of Fitness.

One thing you find with the 'habit but no results' person is that they are no longer growing with exercise. They are doing the same thing day in day out, they don't challenge themselves in ways that deliver the results they want, and while they can be happy that they are moving they are missing out on experiencing the full rewards that come when you are thriving with fitness. This person is a classic example of 'good being the enemy of great'.

For you to stay in the thriving lane it's important you catch yourself when you are falling out of using the Circle of Fitness process. You are looking for that moment where you have forgotten to do a step in the process, or after you have finished a circle loop you create a gap before you do the 'assess' step again.

If you catch yourself falling away aim to get back on track asap!

There are two things to do if you find yourself in this position:

1. **Assess if you want to stay on the same path:**
   Sometimes the path we put ourselves on isn't the right
   path and unfortunately for some people this means they
   fall completely away from fitness. If you are in this place
   assess if you want to stay on the current path. If you do,
   spend some time determining what is taking you out of
   your Circle of Fitness and then develop strategies to get
   back on track. If you find that your current path is not for
   you then try the next option.

2. **Start a new Circle:** This requires you to dig deeper than
   you did in assessing whether you want to stay on the
   same path. You need to determine why your last plan
   didn't work. It may be that you set the wrong challenge
   based on the current demands within your life, it may
   be that the challenge was too much of a step up, or
   it could be that it was too easy. By creating a deeper
   understanding at this point you'll be able to make better
   choices around the next circle you move into.

Ultimately at the end of this process you will have a perfect
challenge that will motivate you to keep growing your fitness
journey. Now you can get back on track and start working through
your next journey.

The Circle of Fitness is also a powerful tool to use when it's time
to change the type of exercise you do. When I was doing Ironman
I was in love with the sport. I loved training for hours every day
and I loved facing the massive physical challenges the sport put
in front of me. I was definitely in a place where I was thriving.

After six years and having completed my Ironman goal, I was
starting my next Circle of Fitness journey. In my assessment phase
I realised that I wanted to have time for other things in my life and
Ironman was no longer going to fit. This assessment phase helped
me realise that it was time for me to move on from Ironman and
find fitness goals that were more realistic. I needed to shift my
exercise life to one where I would only train for 8-14 hours a week

rather than 20-35 hours.

Once I gave up Ironman so many people asked me if I missed the sport and in some ways I did but it was easy for me to let go because the process the Circle of Fitness took me through helped me see that this sport no longer worked for my life.

There are many people in the Ironman world who stopped thriving with the sport years ago but they are still doing the same thing day in and day out because it's the habit they have. By letting go of Ironman I was able to put my focus in other areas, areas where I've learnt new skills and grown myself way more than what would have been possible if I had just kept doing that sport.

By always being aware of where you are within the Circle of Fitness you can catch when it's time to reassess or if it's time for you to make big changes in your fitness journey. This will help you stay in the place where you are thriving more often.

STRATEGY #4: Evolve the Circle of Fitness and make it your own

The Circle of Fitness is a simple framework you can work with to keep you in the right place with fitness. Like all successful frameworks I recommend you follow it to a tee but at the same time how you apply it will be something you will take ownership of and evolve.

For example, in the 'assess' phase you may like to get a journal and have a deep writing session where you explore some tough questions, or you may plan a meeting with one of your mentors so they can help you find your answers. What you are aiming to learn is how you work best in each phase of the Circle and as time goes on you want to evolve your own process.

The deeper the understanding you have of how you work, the easier it will be for you to grow and evolve. This will be so valuable to you and it will enable you to grow to levels that you never thought possible.

I can 100% guarantee that if you keep the Circle of Fitness as a tool you use regularly you will have a lifetime love of fitness. What

I love even more is that you can't even see what your future will look like with fitness because there will be different challenges, different movements, different communities and people, and different areas of growth. This is so exciting because it means you are going to have a life that is full of experiences where your health and fitness will always be in a great place. This is a life worth living.

Mindsets to practise in Baby Step 9

- I will always use the Circle of Fitness in my life, which means I can always thrive with fitness.

- I will always catch when I'm falling away from the Circle of Fitness and if this happens I will instantly commit to reassessing.

- I will continually evolve my Circle of Fitness process.

Workbook for Baby Step 9

Because we are now addressing your long-term fitness journey, the workbook for this Baby Step is the process you can use when you start applying the Circle of Fitness.

In each of the steps of the Circle I'll give you some questions to work through. My questions are only a guide—you may find better ones that work for you.

Step 1: Assessment

What did I learn from the last Circle I completed?

Where am I currently at in each of these areas?:

- Skills (around the movement you are focusing on)

- My mental game

- The social side of my movement

- My life balance

- My level with my movement (for example you could be a grade 3 cyclist)
- My relationship with my mentors
- Other areas that are important to me

Step 2: Decide where you want to grow next

- Based on my assessment and the time and energy I have to commit, where do I want to develop myself over the next period of time?
- What would it take to achieve this growth?
- Is this realistic?
- Success with this growth would mean...
- How could this development evolve me as an overall person?
- How will this development help me move towards my higher-level goals?

Step 3: Create the challenge

- Based on where I'm aiming to grow, what is the right challenge for me to aim for?
- Who can help me and how can they help me?
- How do I make sure I get a plan that gives me the wisest path forward?
- What do I have to give up to achieve this challenge?
- What hurdles do I need to be aware of on this path?
- Why is this challenge the right challenge for me?
- Outside of my movement, what can this challenge teach me about myself?

Step 4: Go on your journey

- How do I stick to my plan as much as possible?

- How can I become a master of catching when I'm falling away from my plan? And when I do, how do I make sure I get back to it asap?

- Who will be the people that will help me be successful and what do I need to communicate with them?

- What can I do to make sure I get the best out of myself?

- How can I keep reminding myself that this challenge is good for me?

- Why is this challenge the right challenge for me?

Step 5: Face your challenge

- What attitude will best serve me with this challenge?

- Other than the result, what will success in this challenge look like?

- What have my previous experiences taught me that I can use in this experience?

- When it gets tough, what will I do to increase the chance of success?

- What do I enjoy about this challenge?

- Where can I grow as a person through this challenge?

Step 6: Celebrate

- Celebrate in a way that feels right to me

- Celebrate the whole process

Step 7: Learn and reflect

- How can I make sure I do the work that is needed around learning and reflecting?

- What process will I use to make sure I get the most out of this time? For example, what questions will I ask myself?

- Who needs to be a part of this process?

- What time frame after my challenge should this be completed by?

- How do I make sure I understand what my future development looks like?

Success in this step equals:

- You will have the ability to understand and apply the Circle of Fitness to your life.

- You will have practised the Circle of Fitness for 12 months.

- You will be experiencing a thriving place with fitness and you'll know how to get to that place more often.

- You will have trust that you can have exercise in your life for the long term.

- You will continue to evolve with exercise for the long term.

Imagine...

Imagine you have consistently used the Circle of Fitness process for over 12 months and through that you have achieved fitness growth which means you are continually thriving with exercise. Imagine the benefits you will experience and how much you have evolved through this journey. You are not only a fitter and healthier person, you are experiencing a higher level of self.

This is what the Circle of Fitness can do. Make the commitment to it and you will achieve more than you can imagine.

Share your completion of the Circle of Fitness

Once you have completed your first Circle of Fitness share it to our social pages.
Use hashtag #circleoffitnesscompleted

To join our social pages go to:
www.passionaboutexercise.com/social

Remember you can sign up for the Passion for Exercise course by going to:
www.passionaboutexercise.com/course

Chapter 12

How you can change your world in powerful ways

When I was around 18 years old there was a basketball coach in New Zealand called John Dybvig. John was an outspoken American man who wasn't shy of sharing his opinion on all topics of sport which helped him get a lot of airtime on radio and TV shows. If you aren't a Kiwi, one thing you need to know about New Zealanders is that we tend to be a relatively understated culture when it comes to the public showing of emotion. When one of our top sports stars scores an important try or goal or wins a big game they celebrate, but with measured control. This is one of the reasons why John was so popular with the media; he was brash and he didn't care.

In the 90s, basketball was a very small sport in New Zealand. It's grown a lot since then but at that time the majority of New Zealanders wouldn't have been able to name one representative in the New Zealand men's basketball team. The knowledge and participation in the female game was even smaller and this is what makes John Dybvig so interesting. He was the coach of the New Zealand women's basketball team. This man got just about as much radio and TV time as the leading rugby and netball coaches (the most popular sports at that time), and he coached a very unknown team in a very small sport. Before John turned up, the New Zealand women's basketball team would have been lucky to get one or two news segments on the major news networks every year. Once John arrived, suddenly basketball got a lot more attention.

A few years after John retired I listened to an interview with him; it was looking back over his career. The interviewer asked him why he had always been so outspoken and brash in the media and I thought that he would talk about the difference between New Zealand and American culture, but his answer showed a deeper insight. He said that if you love a sport, part of your job is to grow the sport. He always knew that his strong opinions would get him in the media and that gave him the ability to promote and grow the game of basketball. John didn't just see his job as being a great basketball coach, he saw it as getting more people loving the game itself.

I don't know how much credit we can give to John Dybvig for the massive growth of basketball in New Zealand since the 90s. I'm sure the global growth of the sport has played a big part too but he can definitely take some credit.

This leads us into the next Baby Step, but before I reveal it I want to share one more thing.

I want you to think about influence for a second. Influence is an interesting thing. The dictionary defines it as 'the capacity to have an effect on the character, development, or behaviour of someone or something'.

When you think about your life, how many people have influenced you? Who has influenced you in powerful ways and who has influenced you in ways that have worked against you? When you think about the people who had a positive influence, what did they do to create this? Why did you want to listen to them?

Do you think you influence others? If so, how?

The next thing I want you to think about is inspiration. Inspiration comes in many forms. I remember watching the documentary *Free Solo* which was about Alex Honnold becoming the first person to perform a free solo climb of El Capitan in Yosemite National Park in America. This documentary was intensely draining, I felt like I was climbing the cliff myself! What Alex did was unbelievable and I was inspired by what Alex had achieved.

There are lots of examples of human feats that give us the energy spark that inspiration delivers; sporting achievements, artistic performances, or someone overcoming adversity. But there's a problem with inspiration—often it doesn't lead to any change.

After I watched *Free Solo* I didn't take up free climbing. Looking back I don't think I changed anything in my life as a result of watching this documentary that had such an impact on me. I was inspired but I stayed the same. Unfortunately this happens a lot. We have moments where we are inspired by others but it doesn't drive us to action change.

I think one of the main reasons for this is because we are often inspired by people who are well above our ability. When Serena Williams hits a game-winning shot I am inspired but I don't think to myself, 'I can be like Serena and win the Australian Open'. What they achieve is out of reach for most of us.

When you do a Google search for inspirational people, names that come up include: Michael Jordan, Billie Jean King, Neil Armstrong, Mother Teresa, and Nelson Mandela. They are certainly inspirational but most people will think, 'I can't be like Michael Jordan'.

This type of inspiration is noneffective. Inspiration is meant to motivate action to help someone move forward in life and while it's nice to have these moments, I want you to understand the most powerful inspiration of all.

When we first started helping people achieve their 5km running goal we discovered the best marketing tool of all time—*make sure people actually achieve the result*. When people signed up for our running programme we made a commitment to them that they will run 5km because we were good at what we did and the programme was achievable.

As a business owner I made sure I had a good marketing budget and as the business grew after every sales period we would do a review of how people had found out about us. The money I had spent on advertising had brought people in but the number one sales generator for us by a country mile was referrals.

It seemed like everyone who ran 5km with us would bring two or three more people to the group and when I asked the people who had been referred why they decided to join, this is when I truly understood inspiration. They would say things like, 'I saw my workmate who had never done exercise before achieve a fitness goal that I would love to achieve and I thought to myself "if they can do it, so can I". I started to understand that our total beginners who went on to run 5km became an inspiration to the people in their lives.

While inspiration from people way above our level of ability definitely has a place in our lives, real inspiration happens when someone just like us creates change. It might be your non-exercising friend who goes on to complete their first triathlon, or it could be a work colleague who makes a breakthrough with their weight loss, or a friend who pulls back from drinking too much. When people like you actually create change it opens you up to the possibility that you can change too. You can see yourself at the same level and have an 'If they can do it I can do it too' moment.

This was why we kept getting referrals and the thing that I loved the most was telling those people that they were a fitness inspiration. Here was someone who hadn't done any exercise for years, went on their own 5km running journey and achieved a goal they were proud of and now they were inspiring others. You could see them being proud of themselves when they realised this.

Here's the thing; if you have been working through this book, have gone through this journey and have completed all of the Baby Steps, you too are an inspiration. The people in your life who have seen you do this—witnessed your growth and achievements—may be thinking to themselves, 'If they can do it, so can I'.

Stop and think about this for a moment—*you are an inspiration to the people in your life.*

Your actions are opening them up to possibility, the possibility that they can do this too, they can achieve growth that can change their life. Michael Jordan has nothing on you.

You have influence. You have gone through a journey of change and have experienced it first hand. You have credibility and people will listen to you. Credibility gives you this influence.

This is where your journey gets powerful and in many ways will be the most rewarding part.

If you become an inspiration to people in your world, and you have influence on these people, imagine what you can do with it.

I want you to have the understanding that John Dybvig had, with this inspiration and influence you can help more people love movement. Your own growth journey is an amazing thing but this gets multiplied when you help others grow in the same way.

This leads to our last Baby Step.

Baby Step 10: Help others learn to love and grow with exercise

If you have gone through the journey of this book and are now at a place where you have achieved your first fitness goals you will be experiencing the benefits that come with this which may include:

- You are fitter and healthier.
- You have more energy.
- You have found a passion for movement.
- You have created friendships and are a part of a community.
- You have grown in ways you would have never thought possible.
- You have had new experiences.
- You have achieved goals you are proud of.

- You have changed how you see yourself around exercise.

- You will feel better about yourself.

- You will probably be doing better in other areas of your life.

I could go on and on, there are so many benefits that come with getting to this point.

Take a moment to reread all of those benefits. Imagine if you could give those to someone else, it could be a friend, a workmate, a family member, or a young person in your life who isn't currently active.

I fundamentally believe that life is better with exercise in it. You have the ability to help others get to this place. That's what this Baby Step is all about.

Challenge for Baby Step 10

To help at least one person be successful with their fitness journey. You can choose one person, a group of friends or a few of your work colleagues. All you need to know is that at the end of this period of time someone or some people in your life will have had a successful exercise experience.

Rules for Baby Step 10

RULE #1: Make a commitment to the person/people you choose

We have all had people in our lives who are the 'fly-by-nighters'. They talk a big game about being there for you and supporting you no matter what, but when you really need them they are nowhere to be seen.

Then you have that person who is always there for you. They stand beside you in times of celebration and lift you up and support you in times of need. These people have a commitment to your relationship that is unconditional. By having them in your world you have a support person who helps you navigate through life in a healthier way.

For a lot of people, starting a fitness journey is a very vulnerable thing to open up to. Having the support of someone like you will be valuable in so many ways but you can't be half committed; you have to be there for the whole journey.

By deciding to do this Baby Step you are making a commitment that you are going to stick it out no matter what. When the struggles come, you will not give up on them. There may be times when you need to get up early and meet them for a session because you know they need you to help with motivation—you will do this because you know that will make a difference. There will be times when they have doubts—you will listen and guide them because you know if they get through this moment they will stay on track.

I'm not saying you have to hold their hand through every single step of their journey, but commit to showing a level of support that will help them through to the end of their first fitness win.

RULE #2: Be their support crew and cheerleader

You are going to have an important role in this person's life but I'm not asking you to be everything for them. See your job as a support crew and cheerleader. They will have many people around them to help them be successful on their fitness journey, like you did. Coaches, mentors, their family and friends network, the community they find around the movement they enjoy, and other training partners. All of these different people will offer different support to this person's journey, but your number one job is to be their support crew/cheerleader. Support and cheer is the affirmation you want to keep at the forefront of your mind when doing this Baby Step.

RULE #3: Let them have their own experience

Years ago I realised I was doing something that was ruining a special moment in someone else's life. In the world of group fitness one of the early highlights you can achieve is being a workshop presenter. This is where you get to present a track in front of all of your peers and are an example of how it should be done, you are seen as a role model. When I first became a workshop presenter I was so proud of myself. I remember seeing the pamphlet with my name on it and having a 'this is me' moment. After my first workshop presentation I kept getting asked back to do it over and over again.

A few years later I had climbed further up the ladder of my career and being a workshop presenter was just another thing I did and while I still respected the opportunity it was no longer something special to me.

One workshop I was working with an instructor who was presenting for the first time. I could see they were nervous, excited and really wanted to do a good job. The day before the presentation we caught up for a practice and it was in this session I did something that, looking back now, I'm disappointed in myself about. I was talking to the new presenter about how it was easy, that I didn't even have to do much prep for it, and that being a presenter wasn't that much of a challenge. I was being a dork. You could see as I was talking that the excitement was draining out of their face. I let this person down.

Luckily I did learn from this. I learnt that even though this person was new to this experience and wasn't at the same level as me at that moment, it was an exciting moment in their development and it was my job to nurture this excitement. I learnt that I wanted to encourage their opportunity to perform at the next level, to appreciate that this is a challenge for them and my job is to help them be their best. I also learnt that I can teach by doing, that my example can show them what the higher level looks like.

Unfortunately a lot of people who are at a higher level just want to show off (like I did) when they are dealing with people who are just starting out on their journey. That is not about helping others, it's about ego.

We also need to be mindful of not pre-empting their experience. You see this often with people who have done marathons. When they talk to someone who is at the beginning of their running journey they tell them what they are going to experience, and they continue to do this every step of the way. This isn't in a guiding or nurturing way, they just want to talk about their own experience.

Even though you may know what they are going to go through—the hurdles they will come up against, the highs they will experience—you need to let them have their own experience. Sure, there will be times when you need to guide them though but let them have the moments that come with their journey. Remind yourself that you are their support crew/cheerleader on their journey of self discovery. Embrace and feed their growth and know that by doing this you'll be helping them more effectively.

Strategies to use in Baby Step 10

STRATEGY #1: Choose someone that you feel is ready for this journey

This Baby Step is a fun project that has the potential to give you rewards that are so fulfilling, not to mention the impact you can have on someone else's life that could be life changing! As this is the first time you have done this we want to set you up for success so you need to choose the right person to work with. This person will be someone who has shown interest in wanting to make change and whom you feel is ready to take the next steps forward with their exercise.

You may know someone that you feel needs this more than others. They may be extremely unhealthy and unfit and may seem like the obvious choice but if they aren't interested in doing this, you'll have a much harder job helping them. Don't get me wrong, I want you to help as many people as possible make shifts in their lives but as this is your first time helping someone with their fitness journey, I want you to gain the understanding of how to successfully help people in their journey so you'll be better prepared for those who may present a harder challenge.

A good way to identify the person you are going to work with is to choose someone that has shown interest in the journey you have been on. They may have asked you questions about what you have learnt, given you compliments on the change you have created, or even have straight out asked you for help. Often their interest in your journey is them reaching out for help, it's just that they need you to offer first.

When you approach them, let them know about this book and the project you are working on. Let them know that you want to be their support person and cheerleader and that you are on their team and together you are about to go on a cool ride.

STRATEGY #2: Give them this book

By going through this journey you now understand that this book can help beginners be successful in finding a love for exercise. As you know I've created a clear and achievable step-by-step framework that allows people to focus on a growth pathway. By giving them this book you can use this framework to create success for them. You will be able to answer their questions based on your experiences and you'll be able to give them tips along the way.

STRATEGY #3: Determine how the relationship will work

Set an understanding of how the relationship will work from the start; how often you will communicate, if you will train together, what they can do when they are struggling with motivation, and so on. Aim to catch up for coffee before you start and set a plan in place. This may seem like an awkward conversation to have but if you commit to doing it, it will be worth its weight in gold.

STRATEGY #4: Be a great accountability partner

One of the most popular things people say they need when they get someone to guide and support them on a growth journey is accountability. Accountability to someone else seems to be a good motivation tool but it can get tricky.

Let's say you are the support person and you know the person you are working with has missed their last three sessions. You get in contact to check in with them and help them to ensure they turn up and do their next session. A few days later you learn that they missed that session as well. This is when it can get challenging. A gap in the relationship can start to form and contact between you both can get difficult. The elephant in the room is ever-present at this point.

If this happens, remind yourself that they wanted your help and they wanted you to keep them accountable but you don't want to make them feel guilty. I guarantee they have enough of that going on just through their own thoughts and feelings. Your job at this point is to just get them to do their next session and communicate that you are supporting them to find the easiest way for them to do this.

Let them know you are keeping them accountable because you care and that you made a commitment and you want to work with them to help them get over this hurdle. This open 'team' approach will help them see that you are on their side and you aren't doing this to make them feel guilty—you are there to help them succeed.

Determining how the relationship will work should be a part of the conversation you have at the start.

STRATEGY #5: Create a 'check in' system for your own planning

One of my best mates, Duncan, never forgets a birthday or anniversary. Often I'll get a text on my wedding anniversary from Duncan before I have even acknowledged it with my wife, Jo! You know that Duncan really cares about you as a mate because he always remembers to acknowledge the special moments.

Duncan's diary alerts make sure he never forgets these important dates and the little bit of time he spends creating these reminders has a massive return for him because every time a friend of Duncan's gets a message on an important day they feel that they are important and that they are connected with him.

Because Duncan cares, he has a system that keeps him on top of the important days and this is what you want to do. Most of us have busy lives and there are so many things we intend to do but they just get forgotten. For you to be a good support person you don't want to go a couple of weeks where you missed checking in. Create a 'check in' system for your support relationship. It could be as simple as setting an alarm to go off on your phone once or twice a week as a reminder. When the alarm goes off send a text, give them a call or plan a catch up.

By having this system in place you will always be showing support and reinforcing your commitment. This will build a stronger relationship and help them stay on their path.

STRATEGY #6: Be great at catching and reinforcing their wins and growth

When I was doing Ironman I had a performance I was really proud of. I was racing at Ironman New Zealand and I had one of the best runs in the whole field. When I got to the finish line I was over the moon with my result and I was super proud of my run because I had worked hard on this area over the last year. The hours of hard work had paid off and it delivered a high level of satisfaction because I knew I had grown.

A couple of weeks later I was at my local swimming pool and I bumped into Scott Molina. Scott is an absolute legend in the triathlon world, he's won the Ironman World Championship and in the 80s his nickname was The Terminator because he seemed to win just about every race he entered. When I bumped into Scott he told me that I had absolutely nailed it, that there were much higher level guys who didn't perform at my level in that race and that he was proud of me.

This was such a powerful moment in my life. I had worked hard to achieve growth as a runner and when I was tested I stepped up to a new level. I was already feeling proud of myself but then a man I had so much respect for gave me praise—that made me feel even better. I left my conversation with Scott feeling motivated to find my next level as an athlete.

A big part of being a great supporter and cheerleader is catching your person's wins. When you see them, acknowledge them through words that reinforce they have done well and why you are impressed by their growth. This is a gift that will stay with them, keep them motivated and will help them see that they are progressing. Remember, you can never do too much of this, as long as it's deserved, always catch and reinforce their wins.

Strategy #7: Learn how to get better at being a great support person

Part of your journey in this Baby Step is to learn how to be a great support person to someone else. I've shared ideas in this step but a lot of your learning will come from the experience you've had. Aim to evolve how you go about being a support person, learn what works and what doesn't. You could even invest some time learning about techniques that coaches and mentors use to bring out the best in others.

This Baby Step is about helping one person in your life but my ultimate aim is for you to help many people in the years ahead. The more you can learn about how to bring the best out in others the more impact you are going to have on the world. Challenge yourself to learn more about this side of your journey. You can do this by reading books, watching videos from leading coaches and mentors or even talking to leaders you know and asking them what they do to create success for others.

Strategy #8: Enjoy it for yourself

Although this is about helping someone else, it should also be enjoyable for you. Catch and embrace the moments where you get something back from this experience. These will include when you feel proud of your person, when you have a shared experience, when you help them overcome a hurdle they face or even when you have a moment of human connection. This has the potential to be hugely rewarding. Embrace every moment and enjoy what this brings to your life.

STRATEGY #9: Be part of their big day

If your person has a goal day like an event or race, be part of it! You could be their support crew, their cheerleader, the person who high-fives them when they have finished their challenge—or all of the above! You don't want to miss this because I guarantee that you will feel like a proud parent as you watch them achieve this goal that they may never have thought possible. It will be a moment you will remember forever and you can be proud of yourself because you are a big part of why this person is experiencing this special moment.

Mindsets to practise for Baby Step 10

- My job is to be the ultimate support person and cheerleader.

- I will guide them but also let them have their own experience.

- This experience is teaching me how to become great at supporting others.

- I need to catch and praise them for their wins along the way.

- I'll keep seeing how I'm making a difference in someone else's life.

While this Baby Step is about helping one person have a successful exercise experience, my ultimate aim is for you to be a person who helps many people learn to have a love of exercise and there are many ways this can happen.

If you live and share my philosophy that if people get into a successful fitness habit and be like John Dybvig and spread the word to help others learn to love exercise, your reach will go beyond what you think is possible.

Imagine if the person you help with this Baby Step then goes on to help someone else, and that person helps someone else, and so on and so on. Imagine the impact you will have on the world. It's mind blowing stuff.

You can also help more people through becoming more involved in your fitness community. Become a person who helps to build your community and welcome more people into your world.

Ultimately I want you to see yourself as a leader, a leader that has the ability to help others in ways that will help them achieve things they never thought possible, to grow and to become fitter and healthier people. How you go about doing this is your journey but I can guarantee that by doing this you will live a life that is full in so many important ways. You'll not only be a person who has a lifetime love of fitness, you will also have a massive impact on your world.

Workbook for Baby Step 10

This workbook is designed to help you find the right person to help and set a good plan in place when it comes to working together on their journey.

1. Who is the right person to go on this journey with?

2. What are the first steps I need to take with this person?

3. What do we both need to establish about how this relationship will work?

4. What is my role in their journey and how can I make sure I can be my best with this?

5. What is the commitment I'm looking to make with them?

6. What will I do if they are struggling?

7. How will I boost them up along the way?

8. What part of their experience can I share with them?

9. How do I stay focussed on letting them have their own journey?

10. How can I develop myself as a mentor/leader?

Success in this step equals:

- You will have supported and guided someone to achieve their first fitness goal.

- You will have seen this person break through their own barriers.

- You will have learnt lessons about how to be a good leader/mentor.

- You will have experienced the amazing benefits of helping someone else grow.

- You will be open to helping more people moving forward and will be excited about doing this.

- You will have reinforced your own health and fitness identity.

- You will feel like you are making the world a better place.

Imagine...

Through your own journey you are now the inspiration to someone you know and they are now asking you for help and support so they can follow your footsteps and bring exercise into their life. You do this and they are now successfully starting their own exercise journey. Imagine how you feel as you watch their progress and see them experience the great things that come with

HOW YOU CAN CHANGE YOUR WORLD IN POWERFUL WAYS

being regularly active. Then, think about how proud you will be on their challenge day. You will be their cheerleader and you will also be proud of yourself because you have been their inspiration, support and an intrinsic part of their journey.

This is all in front of you. You are about to help change someone's life.

Share a picture of you and the person you are going to help

Go to our social page and share a photo of yourself and the person your are helping to bring exercise into their life. Make sure you add the hashtag #myexercisefriend

To join our social pages go to:
www.passionaboutexercise.com/social

Remember you can sign up for the Passion for Exercise course by going to:
www.passionaboutexercise.com/course

Chapter 13

Final words

I want to speak to two different groups of people here—those who have read the book but haven't started their journey yet, and those who have completed the Baby Steps and have reached the end of this journey.

For those who haven't started their journey

This is an important moment for you. It could be a moment where you put down this book and it will be forgotten, just another book you have read but didn't act upon. Or, this can be the moment where you make a change and start your journey. The fact that you are reading this means you have come to the end of the book and have connected with the Baby Step framework. Make this moment the time where you start your journey.

Don't over-complicate it—go back to Baby Step 1, reread that step and just work on that challenge. That's all you need to do. Rereading and setting yourself up to act upon the challenge in Baby Step 1 will probably be only 30 minutes of your time. This 30 minutes will have a massive return for you as it will get you started. From there you will start building your wins and your momentum which will lead you back to this very page but this time you will be reading the other paragraphs—my words to those who have completed this journey and now have a lifetime love of exercise.

Thirty minutes, give yourself that. Your health and fitness are worth it.

For those who have completed the Baby Steps

Wow, you have done it! I hope you have connected with our world throughout your journey (and hopefully I have connected with you along the way) and have shared your experiences. You have achieved something that so many people aren't even willing to try.

While I'm sure it's been a massively positive experience, one where you have gained so much along the way, I know you have put a lot of effort in and I'm proud of you. I'm also excited about the future you have in front of you. This is a future where your love of exercise will provide growth, fulfilment, new experiences, new relationships, deeper understanding of yourself and so, so much more.

Use your journey to keep inspiring others to find the love that you have found and together we can make a difference to our world. Thanks.

Thank you for taking the time to read this book. I hope I've given you the tools and strategies for you to create important change in your life.

Remember you can get my course

If you haven't started your journey and would love more support, accountability, deeper insight, and a guide to hold your hand through the process sign up for my Passion for Exercise course. It will be the best thing you can do to help yourself on this journey.

You can sign up for the Passion for Exercise course by going to:
www.passionaboutexercise.com/course

About the Author

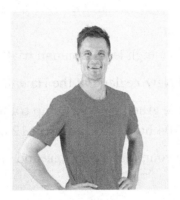

Bevan has always been driven by the question: 'What does it take to create a lifetime love of fitness where people experience all the benefits of a healthy lifestyle choices?'. Through his own experiences and the experiences of helping others, he has learnt valuable lessons and insights into what it takes to create a love of fitness so that movement and exercise become a necessary and rewarding part of our daily lives.

Since 1999, Bevan has been a world leading fitness professional, a high level athlete and continues to inspire and motivate people across the globe. He has achieved top awards and recognition within his industry and is recognised and respected throughout the sports and fitness world.

Bevan has achieved a lot during his career as a fitness professional, an athlete and a content creator:

As a fitness professional:

- 3 x National Fitness Instructor of the year
- Travelled the globe training other fitness professionals
- Represented Les Mills as an International Master Trainer
- Created New Zealand's most successful running group training business
- Teaches and leads over 1000 people a week to discover and evolve their love of exercise

As an athlete:

- Completed as a high level Ironman triathlete
- Represented New Zealand at the Hawaii Ironman
- Completed the gruelling Epic Camp training camp, where he did over 104 hours of exercise in 12 days
- Competed in countless marathons and endurance cycling events

As a content creator:

- Has three highly successful and respected fitness podcasts
- Has been a regular writer for his country's leading newspapers
- The author of a top selling fitness book 'The Fitness Attitude'
- A mentor and personal coach for clients around the world

While Bevan is proud of all his achievements both personally and what he has helped others achieve, he is most proud of what he and his team are doing to help non-exercisers bring exercise into their lives with his Get up to Five beginner running programme. Bevan and his team have guided, supported and trained thousands of non-exercisers to run 5km and have helped them develop a love for movement.

'When you help someone that isn't exercising discover the love of movement and regular exercise, you see them create massive shifts. I fundamentally believe that your life is better if you have exercise in it and I see it as my job to get as many people moving as possible'.

– Bevan James Eyles

You can find Bevan at www.bevanjameseyles.com

Made in the USA
Middletown, DE
17 February 2024

49942552R00146